Authors

Dana F. Oakes, BA, RRT-NPS
Educational Consultant

Formerly:
Director of Respiratory Care
V.A. Medical Center
Washington, D.C.

Director of Clinical Education
Respiratory Care Program
Columbia Union College
Tacoma Park, Maryland

Sean P. Shortall, RRT-NPS, RPFT
Clinical Application Specialist

Formerly:
Clinical Education Coordinator
Respiratory Medicine Department
Eastern Maine Medical Center
Bangor, Maine

Critical Care Educator
Dartmouth-Hitchcock Medical Center
Lebanon, New Hampshire

Scot N. Jones, BA, RRT-ACCS
Director of Clinical Education
Broward College
Coconut Creek, Florida

Formerly:
Supervisor, Respiratory Care
Vidant Medical Center
Greenville, North Carolina

Table of Contents

at-a-glance

Chapter

Ventilator Indications and Goals 1

Parameters and Operation................................. 2

Modes of Ventilation 3

Initial Settings.. 4

Assessment and Trouble-Shooting 5

Ventilator Graphics 6

Equations 7

Management... 8

Noninvasive Ventilation..................................... 9

Diseases and Disorders 10

Effects and Cautions 11

Discontinuation/Weaning................................. 12

Appendix / Index .... A

Turn to Page 1 of each chapter for a
DETAILED TABLE OF CONTENTS

ISBN 978-0-932887-47-4

RespiratoryBooks
A Division of Health Educator Publications, Inc.
476 Shotwell Road
Suite 102, PMB 161
Clayton, NC 27520

RespiratoryBooks.com

Important Disclaimer:

The Authors and Publisher has exerted every effort to ensure that the clinical principles, procedures, and practices described herein are based on current knowledge and state-of-the-art information available from acknowledged authorities, texts, and journals. Nevertheless, they cannot be considered absolute and universal recommendations. Each patient situation must be considered individually. The reader is urged to check the package inserts of drugs and disposable equipment and the manufacturer's manual of durable equipment for indications, contraindications, proper usage, warnings, and precautions before use. The Author and Publisher disclaim responsibility for any adverse effects resulting directly or indirectly from information presented in this book, undetected errors, or misunderstandings by the readers.

Assistant Editors

James K. Stoller, MD, MS, FCCP
Professor and Chairman
Education Institute
Jean Wall Bennett Professor of Medicine
Lerner College of Medicine
Cleveland Clinic
Cleveland, Ohio

Angella T. Crane, BA
Respiratory Therapy Assistant
Indiana University Health West Hospital

Respiratory Therapy Student (2015)
Ivy Tech Community College
Indianapolis, Indiana

Michael W. Hess, BS, RRT
Respiratory Therapist
United States Department of Veterans Affairs
Kalamazoo, Michigan

Aaron C. Kulukjian, RCP, RRT-NPS
Respiratory Therapist
Sutter Medical Center Sacramento
Sacramento, California

Joshua Nerren, RRT-NPS, NREMT
Respiratory Therapist
Providence Sacred Heart Medical Center & Children's Hospital
Spokane, Washington

1 Ventilator Indications and Goals

CONTENTS

Indications for Ventilatory Support 1-2
Contraindications to Ventilatory Support 1-3
Acute Respiratory Failure (Types) 1-3
Indications for Invasive Support (Algorithm) ... 1-4
Differential Checklist of Potential Causes of Acute Respiratory Failure 1-5
Clinical Parameters to Determine Ventilatory Need 1-8

ACCP: Objectives of Mechanical Ventilation ... 1-9

Indications for Ventilatory Support

Indications	Description	Examples
Apnea	Absence of breathing	• Cardiac Arrest
Acute Respiratory Failure (ARF)	Inability of a patient to maintain adequate: PaO_2, $PaCO_2$, and, potentially, pH.	• Hypoxemic RF • Hypercapnic RF *See next page for details*
Impending Respiratory Failure	Respiratory failure is imminent in spite of therapies. ***Commonly defined as:*** Pt is barely maintaining (or gradual deterioration) of normal blood gases but with significant WOB.	• Neuromuscular Disease (N-M) • Status Asthmaticus
Chronic Respiratory Failure	Repeated failures after attempts to liberate from the ventilator (extubations, Trach Collar trials, etc.)	**SEVERE**: • Obesity Hypoventilation Syndrome • COPD • Pulmonary Fibrosis
Prophylactic Ventilatory Support	Clinical indication = high risk of respiratory failure. Ventilatory support is instituted to ↓ WOB, minimize O_2 consumption and hypoxemia, reduce cardiopulmonary stress, and/or control airway with sedation.	• Brain injury • Heart muscle injury • Major surgery • Shock (prolonged) • Smoke injury • Trauma (some)
Hyperventilation Therapy	Ventilatory support is instituted to control and manipulate $PaCO_2$ to lower than normal levels.	• Acute head injury (↑ ICP) (not immediately after injury. Review recommendations in disease chapter)

Contraindications to Ventilatory Support

Absolute Contraindications	Relative Contraindications
• Untreated tension pneumothorax (PPV) • Patient's informed refusal (DNI)	• Medical futility * • Patient pain/suffering • Known inability to wean

* *Medical futility*: Consider non-invasive ventilation (NPPV) as an interim measure until ethical considerations are determined.

Two Types of Acute Respiratory Failure

Hypoxemic Respiratory Failure	Hypercapnic Respiratory Failure
Known as: Type I ARF, Lung Failure, Oxygenation Failure, Respiratory Insufficiency	***Known as:*** Type II ARF, Pump Failure, Ventilatory Failure
Definition: The failure of lungs and heart to provide adequate O_2 to meet metabolic needs	***Definition:*** The failure of the lungs to eliminate adequate CO_2
Criteria at sea level: $PaO_2 < 60$ mmHg on $FiO_2 \geq .50$ or $PaO_2 < 40$ mmHg on any FiO_2 $SaO_2 < 90$	***Criteria:*** <u>Acute</u> ↑ in $PaCO_2 > 50$ mmHg or Acutely above normal baseline in COPD with concurrent ↓ in pH < 7.30
Basic Causes: • R-L shunt • V/Q mismatch • Alveolar hypoventilation • Diffusion defect • Inadequate FIO_2	***Basic Causes:*** • Pump failure (drive, muscles, WOB) • ↑ CO_2 production • R-L shunt • ↑ Deadspace

REMINDER: ABG values and other drawn labs should always be interpreted in context of how the patient looks. Decisions to initiate ventilation should not be made simply because a patient has a bad ABG.

Indications for Invasive Ventilation in Adults with Acute Respiratory Failure

1. Apnea or Impending Respiratory Arrest

2. Acute ventilatory insufficiency in neuromuscular disease with any of the following:

- Acute respiratory acidosis
- Progressive decline in VC to less than 10 -15 mL/kg IBW
- Progressive decline in MIF to less than -20 to -30 cm H_2O

3. Acute hypoxemic respiratory failure with the following:

- Tachypnea, respiratory distress and persistent hypoxemia despite high FIO_2 and NPPV with FIO_2
- Or in the presence of any of the following:
  - Acute cardiovascular instability
  - Altered mental status or persistent uncooperativeness
  - Inability to protect the lower airway

4. Acute Exacerbation of COPD with dyspnea, tachypnea, and acute respiratory acidosis plus at least one of the following:

- Acute cardiovascular instability
- Altered mental status or persistent uncooperativeness
- Inability to protect lower airway
- Copious or unusually viscous secretions
- Abnormalities of the face or upper airway
- Progressive respiratory acidosis or other deterioration despite intensive therapy including NPPV

→ **Intubate and Provide Ventilatory Support**

5. Protect airway or manage secretions <u>without</u> an indication for ventilatory support

→ **Intubate**

→ a. Is ETT $\leq$ 7.0 mm with a V_E > 10 L/min?
or
b. Is ETT $\leq$ 8.0 with a V_E > 15 L/min?

- **Yes** → Provide Ventilatory Support
- **No** → Continue to maintain the artificial airway and monitor closely

(Modified from Pierson DJ: *Respiratory Care* 47:3, 249-262, 2002)

Acute Respiratory Failure: A Differential Checklist

Pulmonary	
Acute Airway Obstruction	• Anaphylaxis • Aspiration • Bronchoconstriction • Edema/inflammation • Epiglottitis • Foreign objects • Secretions • Smoke/chemicals • Tracheal/Bronchial malacia or stenosis
Asthma, COPD	• Exacerbation • Late stages
Decreased Lung Tissue functioning (Severe)	• ARDS • Atelectasis • Fibrosis • Pneumonia • Pulmonary Edema • Pulmonary Embolism (PE)
Sleep Disordered Breathing	• Obstructive Sleep Apnea (OSA)
Chest Wall	
Chest Wall	• Flail chest • Kyphoscoliosis / Scoliosis (Severe)/Kyphosis (Severe) • Obesity • Rib fracture • Severe burns
Intra-thoracic	
Intrathorax	• Empyema • Hemothorax • Pleural Disease/Effusions • Pneumothorax

Continued, Next Page

CNS Depression	
CNS	• Cerebral Ischemia, CVA • Drugs: ETOH, anesthetics, barbiturates, cocaine/heroine, methadone, morphine, sedatives, narcotics, etc. • ↑ ICP (hypoxic brain) • Infection • Lesions/tumors • Metabolic alkalosis (CSF) • Obesity Hypoventilation (Pickwickian) • Primary hypoventilation (Ondine's Curse) • Sleep Apnea (Central) • Trauma
Neuromuscular	
Neuro-muscular	• Amyotropic Lateral Sclerosis (ALS) • ***Drugs***: antibiotics, Ca channel blockers, anticholinesterase, curare/non-depolarizers, dexamethonium, methyl alcohol, nerve gases, succinylcholine • Electrolyte imbalance • Guillian-Barré syndrome, Myasthenia gravis • High spinal injury/disease • Multiple sclerosis • Muscular dystrophy • Myotonia • Phrenic nerve injury • ***Poisons/toxins***: botulism, mushrooms, para-quat, petroleum distillates • Poliomyelitis, Polymyositis • Rabies, SLE, Status epilepticus, Tetanus
Cardiovascular	
Cardio-vascular	• Cardiac arrest (↓ CO) • CHF with pulmonary edema • Congenital heart disease • Hypovolemia • Shock • Thromboemboli (Cardiac)

Other	
Other	• Anxiety • Hypothyroidism • Malnutrion / fatigue • Mechanical Ventilation (air-trapping) • Metabolic acidosis • Post-op complications

Clinical Parameters Commonly Used to Determine Ventilatory Need

Parameter*	Normal	MV Indicated
Ventilation		
$PaCO_2$	35-45 mmHg	50-55 mmHg or acute ↑ from pt. baseline (e.g., COPD)
pH	7.35-7.45	< 7.25
V_D/V_T	25-40%	> 60%
Oxygenation		
PaO_2	80-100 mmHg (RA)	< 50 mmHg (RA) < 60 mmHg (50% O_2) < 200 mmHg (100% O_2)
SaO_2	> 95%	< 75%
$PA\text{-}aO_2$	10-25 mmHg (RA)	> 350 mmHg on 100% O_2
$PaO_2\text{-}PAO_2$	0.8-0.9	< 0.15
PaO_2/FiO_2	350-400 mmHg	< 200 mmHg
Q_S/Q_T (shunt)	< 5%	> 20%
Mechanical Capabilities (Mechanics)		
V_T (ideal)	5-8 cc/kg	< 5 cc/kg
f	12-20	< 10 or > 35 prolonged
f/V_T (RSBI)	< 105	> 105
$\dot{V}_E$	5-6 L/min	> 10 L/min
VC (ideal)	60-75 mL/kg	< 15 mL/kg
FEV_1 (ideal)	50-60 mL/kg	< 10 mL/kg
FRC	80-100% predicted	< 50% predicted
MVV	120-180 L/min	< 20 L/min or 2 x $\dot{V}_E$
P_I max (MIP, NIF)	-80 to -100 cmH_20	> -20 cmH_20
Breathing pattern	Normal	Abnormal / Irregular
Intracranial Pressure		
ICP (hyperventilation)	12-15 cmH_20	> 20 cmH_20, impending brainstem herniation, inability to control ↑ ICP's using other methods

* No one parameter or set of parameters has been proven to be an absolute indication of MV. Clinical judgment takes precedence over objective parameters; trends are far more important than absolute values.

Objectives of Mechanical Ventilation *

I. Physiological Objectives

A. Support or Manipulate Pulmonary Gas Exchange

Alveolar Ventilation ($\dot{V}_A$) (e.g., $PaCO_2$, pH)

In most cases, normalize $\dot{V}_A$.

To reduce ICP, $\dot{V}_A$ > normal.

For permissive hypercapnia and acute-on-chronic respiratory failure use adequate, but < normal $\dot{V}A$.

Arterial Oxygenation (e.g., PaO_2, SaO_2, CaO_2)

Achieve acceptable level using acceptable F_IO_2.

In most cases, SaO_2 > 90% or PaO_2 > 60 mmHg.

Seldom used as the only indication for mechanical ventilation, given other techniques available.

B. Increase Lung Volume

End-Inspiratory Lung Inflation

Achieve sufficient lung expansion with every breath (or intermittently)

Used to prevent or treat atelectasis

End-Expiratory Lung Inflation (FRC)

When indicated, achieve, maintain, or ↑ FRC using PEEP therapy.

C. Decrease or Manipulate Work Of Breathing (WOB)

Unload the ventilatory muscles burdened by ↑ Raw or ↓ C_{LT}

II. Clinical Objectives

Reverse Hypoxia (↑PaO_2 and SaO_2 by: ↑ $\dot{V}_A$, ↑ lung volume, and ↓ oxygen consumption)

Reverse Acute Respiratory Acidosis (life threatening)

Relieve Respiratory Distress (intolerable discomfort)

Prevent or Reverse Atelectasis

Reverse Ventilatory Muscle Fatigue (unload ventilatory muscles)

Permit Sedation and/or Neuromuscular Blockade

Decrease Systemic or Myocardial Oxygen Consumption

Reduce Intracranial Pressure (ICP)

Stabilize Chest Wall

*Adapted from ACCP Consensus Conference: Mechanical Ventilation; ***Respiratory Care***, Vol. 38, #12, 1993.

Make It Your Own

Notes Page

2 Parameters and Operation

CONTENTS

Types of Mechanical Ventilation 2-2
Comparison: Full vs. Partial 2-2
Types of Positive Pressure Ventilation 2-3
Comparison: Volume vs. Pressure 2-3

Ventilator Parameters
Volumes 2-4
Rate 2-5
Pressures 2-6
Times 2-9
Flow 2-12
Supplemental Oxygen 2-13
Adjuncts 2-14

Operating Principles
Basic Operating Principles (Volume) 2-17
Basic Operating Principles (Pressure) 2-19
Determinants of Oxygenation 2-20

Types of Mechanical Ventilation

	Full Ventilatory Support	Partial Ventilatory Support
Definition	Ventilator does all the WOB necessary to maintain effective alveolar ventilation.	Patient and ventilator share the WOB necessary to maintain effective alveolar ventilation.
Goals	Achieve **total control** of the patient's ventilatory pattern – patient does not breathe spontaneously or trigger the ventilator.	Achieve only **partial control** of the patient's ventilatory pattern – allow the patient to breathe either spontaneously or trigger (assist) the ventilator.
Indications	Initial ARF – Allowing respiratory muscles to rest, ↓O_2 consumption Need for hyperventilation Patient's disease process (e.g., quadriplegic) Pharmacologic therapy (e.g., paralysis)	*Allow patient to:* • Maintain respiratory muscle tone • Be more synchronous with the ventilator (Synchrony) • Participate in weaning (discontinuation)
Clinical Notes	• This is often referred to as "locking the patient out" and can lead to significant dysynchrony if pt is not adequately sedated and possibly paralyzed • It is not a preferred strategy in most clinical situations • Full support may quickly lead to muscle wasting or atrophy	In most ventilator modes, the clinician determines the balance of WOB provided by the patient vs. the ventilator. **Except: A/C where the ventilator provides most of the WOB (patient can trigger breaths).
Example Modes	• Volume-CMV • Pressure-CMV	**Most Others:** • Volume or Pressure A/C • PRVC or APV • PSV or VSV • APRV

Two Types of Positive Pressure Ventilation

	Volume Ventilation (VV)	Pressure Ventilation (PV)
Other Names	Volume-limited, targeted, controlled, or cycled ventilation.	Pressure-limited, targeted, or controlled ventilation.
Definition	Airflow is delivered by a ventilator that terminates the inspiratory phase of the respiratory cycle after a preset volume is reached	Airflow is delivered by a ventilator to a set inspiratory pressure, which ends the inspiratory phase of the respiratory cycle after a preset time is reached.
Main Charac.	**Volume is set** and remains constant, allowing **pressure to vary**.	**Pressure is set** and remains constant, allowing ***volume to vary***.
Main Advantage	A constant V_T (and/or $\dot{V}_E$) is delivered regardless of changes in patient C or Raw, or ventilator PIP or Pplat.	A constant inflation pressure is delivered regardless of V_T delivery (limits inflation pressure to ↓ risk of alveolar distension). Also has a true decelerating flow.
Major Disadvan.	Alveolar over-distension → ↑ PIP and Pplat if lung condition worsens (i.e., ↑ Raw and/or ↓ C)	Volume delivery (V_T and $\dot{V}_E$ varies as lung condition changes (i.e., either ↑ or ↓ Raw and/or C)
In General	Use Volume if precise $PaCO_2$ regulation is clinical goal, but understand that pressure is relatively unregulated	Use Pressure if overdistension protection or patient-ventilator synchrony is clinical goal, rather than precise $PaCO_2$ regulation

Volume Ventilation vs. Pressure Ventilation

VV	PV
V_T (set); PIP (variable)	**PIP (set); V_T (variable)**
↑ V_T → ↑ PIP + P_{plat} ↓ V_T → ↓ PIP + P_{plat} ↑ C → same V_T (↓ PIP + P_{plat}) ↓ C → same V_T (↑ PIP + P_{plat}) ↑ Raw → same V_T (↑ PIP) ↓ Raw → same V_T (↓ PIP)	↑ PIP → ↑ V_T ↓ PIP → ↓ V_T ↑ C→ same PIP (↑V_T) ↓ C → same PIP (↓V_T) ↑ Raw → same PIP (↓V_T) ↓ Raw → same PIP (↑V_T)

Parameter *(average range)*	Definition	Mechanics	Ventilation Effects	Oxygenation
Volumes				
Minute Volume ($\dot{V}_E$) *(5 – 10 L/min)*	The amount (volume in L) of air moved in and out of lungs in 1 min.	$\dot{V}_E = f \times V_T$ (use average expired V_T in Pressure modes)	$\dot{V}_E \approx \dot{V}_A \approx 1/PaCO_2$	$\dot{V}_E \approx \dot{V}_A \approx PaO_2$
	Too small a $\dot{V}_E \rightarrow$ hypoventilation and possible hypoxemia, Too large a $\dot{V}_E \rightarrow$ hyperventilation Smaller VT may lead to more deadspace and less alveolar (effective) ventilation			
Tidal Volume (V_T) *(5-10 mL/kg)* (6-8 is most common)	Volume of air (mL or cc) delivered to the patient in a single inspiratory breath.	• $V_T = \dot{V}_E / f$ • $V_T = \dot{V}_I \times T_I$ • V_T is commonly set (Volume) or estimated (Pressure) per IBW or disease state in a range. • In Pressure, V_T is variable depending on PIP, PEEP, $\dot{V}_I$, T_I, and patient C and Raw.	($\uparrow V_T \rightarrow \downarrow PaCO_2$) Rate changes, rather than V_T changes, are more commonly employed to regulate $PaCO_2$.	$\uparrow V_T \rightarrow \uparrow \overline{P}aw \rightarrow \uparrow PaO_2$
	Small V_T may result in atelectasis, hypoventilation, and hypoxemia. Large V_T may result in volutrauma, hyperventilation, and $\downarrow$CO. If not compensated for compressible volume some V_T may be undelivered to patient (lost to circuit)			

Parameter *(average range)*	Definition	Mechanics	Ventilation Effects	Oxygenation
Rate				
Ventilator Rate or frequency *(f)* (*12-20 breaths/ min*)	Number of breaths delivered by the ventilator per minute	• $f \times V_T = \dot{V}_E$ • Rate is the main parameter adjusted to change $\dot{V}_E$ and $PaCO_2$ (↑ rate → ↓ $PaCO_2$). • "Normal" rate is highly disease-variable. Faster rates (and smaller V_T's) are commonly used in restrictive disease (short TC). Slower rates are used in obstructive disease (long TC).	$f \times V_T = \dot{V}_E \approx 1/PaCO_2$ TC = time constants (see Equations chapter)	Affects PaO_2 by providing adequate ventilation to the lungs.
	<u>Slow rates</u> may lead to hypoventilation (hypercapnia), hypoxemia, and patient-ventilator asynchrony. <u>Fast rates</u> may lead to hyperventilation (hypocapnia) and/or inadequate T_I and/or T_E, resulting in hypoventilation and/or air-trapping (auto-PEEP) and its accompanying effects.			

Parameter *(average range)*	Definition	Mechanics	Ventilation Effects	Oxygenation
Pressures				
Peak Inspiratory Pressure (PIP or Ppeak) (< 35 cmH_2O)	Highest (peak) proximal airway pressure reached during inspiration.	• Keep PIP < 35 cm H_2O • In Volume – machine V_T, $\dot{V}_I$, PEEP, and patient C_{LT} and Raw determines PIP. • In Pressure: PIP is a set pressure limit • PIP + C_{LT} + Raw = V_T • ↑ PIP → ↑ V_T, Paw, and Palv (except in high Raw where the ↑ pressure is lost to the airway and may not reach the alveoli) • PIP is used to calculate C_{dyn} and Raw.	↑ PIP (V_T) → ↓ $PaCO_2$	↑ PIP ($P\overline{aw}$) → ↑ PaO_2
	<u>Too low a PIP</u> may result in hypoventilation (hypercapnia) and atelectasis. **<u>Too high a PIP</u>** can increase the risk of barotrauma, compromise both ventilation and oxygenation effects, and significantly compromise hemodynamics.			

Parameter *(average range)*	Definition	Mechanics	Ventilation Effects	Oxygenation
Mean Airway Pressure ($\overline{P}aw$) (mPAW) (MAP*)	The mean (average) proximal airway pressure during the entire respiratory cycle.	$\overline{P}aw$ is a function of PIP, PEEP, T_I, T_E, $\dot{V}_I$, and $\dot{V}_I$ waveform. It may be a set parameter on newer ventilators. (PEEP is most direct determinant)	$\overline{P}aw \rightarrow V_T \approx 1/PaCO_2$ $PaCO_2$ $\uparrow$ Paw $\rightarrow \downarrow PaCO_2$	$\overline{P}aw$ is perhaps the major determinant of oxygenation $\uparrow$ Paw $\rightarrow \uparrow PaO_2$
(average depends on other parameters)	**$\overline{P}aw$ Precautions:** Too low a $\overline{P}aw$ may result in hypoventilation and atelectasis. Too high a $\overline{P}aw$ can increase the risk of barotrauma, compromise both ventilation and oxygenation effects, and significantly compromise hemodynamics (mostly by reducing cardiac output).			
Plateau Pressure (Alveolar Pressure) (P_{plat} or P_{alv}) *(< 30 cmH₂O)*	The average alveolar pressure during the inspiratory phase.	P_{plat} is the proximal airway pressure measured during an **inspiratory hold**. It is then assumed to approximate the average (overall) P_{alv} and is used to determine C_{stat} and Raw. P_{alv} is not directly measured.	Generally approximates the effects of PIP.	Generally approximates the effects of PIP.

*Mean Airway Pressure is sometimes abbreviated as MAP, but this is discouraged as this acronym can also be used for Mean Arterial Pressure

Parameter *(average range)*	Definition	Mechanics	Ventilation Effects	Oxygenation
PEEP *($3\text{-}5\ cmH_2O$ is minimum to maintain FRC - referred to as "physiologic")* *($>5\ cmH_2O$ is considered "therapeutic")*	Positive pressure applied during exhalation (a resistance against which the patient passively exhales)	PEEP increases FRC by stabilizing open alveoli to prevent collapse. ↑ **FRC leads to:** 1) ↓ atelectasis → ↓ shunt → ↑ V/Q 2) ↑ C → ↓ WOB 3) ↓ shear force lung injury. PEEP → ↑ Paw → ↑ gas exchange	↑ PEEP may ↑V/Q → ↓$PaCO_2$	↑ PEEP →↑ $\overline{P}aw$ → ↑ V/Q → ↑ PaO_2
	PEEP Precautions - Too low a PEEP when needed may lead to alveolar collapse and ↓ FRC (opposite of mechanics above). Too high a PEEP may lead to over-distension. Over-distension → 1) Air-trapping (auto-PEEP) → volutrauma (and other accompanying effects); 2) ↓C →↑WOB; 3) ↓ venous return → ↓ CO, ↓ UO, and ↑ ICP/↓ CPP; 4) ↑ PVR → ↓ lung perfusion→ ↓ gas exchange; 5) In PV; ↓ (PIP – PEEP) difference → ↓ V_T and ↑ $PaCO_2$			

Types of PEEP

$PEEP_E$ (extrinsic or applied PEEP) = PEEP that is purposely applied by the mechanical ventilator.

$PEEP_I$ (intrinsic, inadvertent, occult, or auto-PEEP) = PEEP that is inadvertently applied by the mechanical ventilator (fast rates/short T_E) and/or patient airway obstruction when flow does not return to zero before the next inspiration starts. Most commonly called auto-PEEP, air-trapping or dynamic hyperinflation. It is PEEP at the alveolar level (intrinsic) and is unintentional and undesirable. (see Chapter 11, Ventilator Effects)

Total PEEP = $PEEP_E + PEEP_I$

Optimal PEEP = Level of PEEP at which maximal oxygenation (increased CaO_2) is obtained with minimal hemodynamic compromise (↓CO) (i.e., O_2 transport = CaO_2 x CO).

Parameter *(average range)*	Definition	Mechanics	Ventilation Effects	Oxygenation
Times				
Inspiratory Time (T_I) (I-Time) *(0.9 – 1.2 sec)*	Duration of the inspiratory phase.	$T_I = T_{tot} - T_E$; $T_I = V_T / \dot{V}_I$ T_I = the I part of the I:E ratio In VV, T_I is often result of $V_T/\dot{V}_I$. In PV, T_I is commonly SET on vent Short T_I's are commonly used in patients with ↓ C (short TC). Longer T_I's are possibly used in patients with ↑ Raw (long TC).	A sufficient T_I is necessary for adequate V_T delivery and, therefore, adequate gas exchange.	Long TI's are used to ↑ $\overline{P}aw$ (↑ T_I → ↑ $\overline{P}aw$ → ↑PaO_2). As T_I ↑, the more time to deliver the V_T, so . . . ↑alveolar distension and ↑ gas exchange.
	T_I Precautions - *Short T_I* (and slow $\dot{V}_I$) may cause ↓ V_T resulting in hypoventilation and hypoxemia. *Long T_I* may cause patient discomfort, patient-ventilator asynchrony and hypoventilation. The longer the T_I the greater the $\overline{P}aw$ and effects on the heart and lungs (see $\overline{P}aw$).			
Expiratory Time (T_E) (E Time) *(1.0 - 5.0 sec)*	Time duration of the expiratory phase. *Most modes use passive exhalation (so expiratory time is not directly set)*	$T_E = T_{tot} - T_I$ T_E = the E part of I:E ratio T_E is often the result of a set T_I (PV), V_T (Vol) and rate (*f*) - rarely set. Longer T_E = more time for lung emptying (esp. important in patients with ↑ Raw).	An adequate T_E is necessary for complete emptying of the lung V_T, and therefore, gas exchange.	Little to no effect on PaO_2 unless T_E is inadequate for lung emptying (causes air trapping = auto-PEEP)

Parameter *(average range)*	Definition	Mechanics	Ventilation Effects	Oxygenation
I:E Ratio (I:E) *(1:1.5 to 1:4)*	Ratio of inspiratory time to expiratory time.	I:E = 1: (T_E/T_I) if E > I (T_E/T_I) : 1 if I > E **I:E ratio may be determined by:** 1) T_I and *f* 2) V_T, $\dot{V}_I$, and *f* 3) Set I:E **Other Relationships:** $I + E = \dot{V}_I / \dot{V}_E$ $\dot{V}_I = \dot{V}_E \times I + E$ $T_I = T_{tot} / I + E$ $T_I \% = 1 / I + E$	An appropriate I:E is necessary for complete filling and emptying of the lung and, therefore, gas exchange.	Larger I:E ratios (larger T_I) →↑ $\overline{P}aw$ and allow greater time for gas distribution, thereby ↑ PaO_2. Inverse ratios (T_I > T_E), to ↑ PaO_2, are generally reserved for patients in severe respiratory failure (high PIP and high F_IO_2) due to the ↑ risks associated with them.
	I:E ratios change with the adjustments of many other parameters. Beware of choosing a desired I:E ratio tc the exclusion of T_I, $\dot{V}I$, and *f*. Equal or inverse ratios (1:1, 2:1, 3:1, etc.) may cause significant ↑ $\overline{P}aw$, patient discomfort, patient-ventilator asynchrony, air-trapping (auto-PEEP), and hemodynamic compromise.			

Parameter *(average range)*	Definition	Mechanics	Ventilation Effects	Oxygenation
Inspiratory Pause (Inflation Hold or Plateau) *(0.5 to 3 sec)*	A delay in the onset of expiration after inspiration is complete.	Inspiratory pause prolongs T_I and ↑ $\overline{P}aw$. May improve gas distribution (recruitment maneuver) Its primary use is to measure static lung compliance or Pplat. It may be applied either by an inspiratory pause control on the ventilator or by briefly occluding expiratory port at end-inspiration.	Little to no effect.	Inspiratory pause → ↑ $\overline{P}aw$ and gas distribution, so may ↑ PaO_2 NOT recommended in clinical practice except as a maneuver to check plateau pressures
	<u>Prolonged T_I</u> and/or prohibiting exhalation may cause patient discomfort, patient-ventilator asynchrony, and possible ↑ $PaCO_2$. Do not use in COPD or patients with expiratory flow limitations. <u>Short T_E</u> may result in air-trapping (auto-PEEP) and its accompanying effects.			
Expiratory Hold (End Expiratory Pause) *(0.5 – 2.0 sec)*	A delay in the onset of inspiration and the prevention of any further exhalation.	At the end of the exhalation time period (just prior to inspiration), the exhalation valve is occluded – preventing any further expiratory airflow and delaying inspiration.	Little to no effect.	Measures auto-PEEP in pt who is not breathing spontaneously

Parameter *(average range)*	Definition	Mechanics	Ventilation Effects	Oxygenation
Flow				
Inspiratory Flow ($\dot{V}_I$) *(40 – 100 L/m)*	The rate at which gas is delivered to the patient during the inspiratory phase.	$\dot{V}_I = V_T / T_I$ Used to provide the desired T_I, I:E ratio, and inspiratory pattern. Goal = $\dot{V}_I \geq$ peak inspiratory demand. Proper $\dot{V}_I = \dot{V}_E \times (I + E)$ Slower $\dot{V}_I$ is used in patients with ↑ Raw and/or poor gas distribution. Slow $\dot{V}_I$ may ↓ PIP and risk of barotrauma in certain diseases. Fast $\dot{V}_I$ may ↓ WOB and improve patient comfort in patients with high inspiratory demand.	An adequate and appropriate $\dot{V}_I$ is necessary for proper ventilation and gas exchange.	$\dot{V}_I$ affects T_I and $\overline{Paw}$ which in turn affects PaO_2.
	Slow $\dot{V}_I$ may not meet the patient's demand (flow-starvation), resulting in ↑WOB, patient discomfort, and possibly hypoventilation. Slow $\dot{V}_I$ results in long T_I and short T_E, leading to patient discomfort and/or air-trapping (auto-PEEP). Fast $\dot{V}_I$ may cause ↑Raw, ↑ PIP, and/or ↓ distribution of ventilation.			
Inspiratory Flow Waveform ($\dot{V}_I$ waveform)	The flow pattern in which inspiratory flow is delivered.	While decelerating flow patterns are popular clinically, some debate exists regarding the "best" waveform		

Parameter *(average range)*	Definition	Mechanics	Ventilation Effects	Oxygenation
Rise Time	The time required to reach the pressure target (PIP) in Pressure modes.	↓ the rise time by ↑ $\dot{V}_I$. ↑ the rise time by ↓ $\dot{V}_I$. Rise time is generally adjusted to "soften" (slow) the initial rapid $\dot{V}_I$.		
	Patient may need a "softer" (slower) rise time for patient-ventilator synchrony. Too slow a rise time may ↑ WOB			
Supplemental Oxygen				
F_IO_2 Goal is to maintain PaO_2 60 – 100 mmHg	The fraction of inspired oxygen delivered to the patient by the ventilator.	Determining factors are to target PaO_2 or SpO_2, PEEP, $\overline{P}aw$, and hemodynamic status. F_IO_2 = decimal (0.21 - 1.0) O_2% = amt of O_2 in % form	None	F_IO_2 determines PAO_2 which in turn affects PaO_2. F_IO_2 1.0 is still recommended before/after suctioning, prior to procedures, etc.
	<u>Low F_IO_2</u> leads to hypoxemia and hypoxia. <u>High F_IO_2</u> may cause O_2 toxicity (lung damage) and intrapulmonary shunting (absorption atelectasis).			

Parameter *(average range)*	Definition	Mechanics	Ventilation Effects	Oxygenation
Adjuncts				
Sensitivity (Inspiratory Trigger Sensitivity)	The level of spontaneous effort (pressure or flow) needed to trigger a machine inspiratory breath.	Sensitivity directly affects patient-ventilator synchrony and interaction. Flow sensitivity is generally preferred due to less WOB required. May need to readjust following changes in PEEP.	Note: Pressure sensitivity: 0.5 to 2.0 cm H_2O below baseline Flow sensitivity: 1 to 3 L/m below baseline	None
Sensitivity (Expiratory Trigger Sensitivity)	% of peak $\dot{V}_I$ at which the ventilator cycles off (I → E)	This is the ventilator's way of determining when a pt is ready to exhale in Pressure Support Ventilation. In a decelerating waveform (as is the case with PSV), as flow slows naturally the threshold % is reached, allowing for transition to exhalation		

Auto-PEEP will affect the patient's ability and effort to trigger the ventilator and must be either eliminated or adjusted for (see Ch 11).
<u>Too sensitive</u> leads to self-cycling (auto-triggering), air-trapping, and potential hyperventilation. <u>Too insensitive</u> promotes increased WOB, atelectasis, patient discomfort, and patient-ventilator asynchrony.

Parameter *(average range)*	Definition	Mechanics	Ventilation Effects	Oxygenation
Sigh [Periodic Hyperinflation] (*1.5 to 2 x normal V_T, every 6-10 minutes*)	The periodic delivery of a larger than normal V_T. *This is thought to replace the normal sigh breath found in non-intubated patients*	Its clinical benefit is unproven. Therapeutic PEEP is commonly recommended instead. **Perhaps consider when:** • Small V_T (< 7 cc/kg IBW) during controlled ventilation • Reexpansion of collapsed lung • Bronchoscopy (during/after) • Some evidence suggests its use in certain neuromuscular disorders	Its use will insignificantly affect $\dot{V}_E$ or $PaCO_2$	May indirectly improve oxygenation through recruitment of alveoli (though questionable)

Parameter *(average range)*	Definition	Mechanics	Ventilation Effects	Oxygenation
Humidification 100% humidity at body temperature; 30 mg H_2O/L absolute humidity; *32 – 37 °C*	The delivery of a heated and humidified gas to the patient.	Prevents water loss from airway. HMEs may be used except when: Secretions are thick, copious and/or bloody. $\dot{V}_E$ > 10 L/min Body temperature < 32°C Expired V_T < 70% delivered V_T		
	Humidity systems should be servo-controlled with temperature readout and alarm (37 ° C). ↓ humidity may result in dried secretions and plugging. Changes in H_2O level of reservoir will change compliance of circuit.			
Mechanical Deadspace (VD_{mech}) *50 to 300 mL of circuit tubing added in 50 mL increments*	Artificial deadspace added between the patient's ET tube and the circuit wye.	Used to keep $PaCO_2$ normal in hyperventilating patients when rate is not controlled. This method is NOT typically used clinically anymore	Added to maintain $PaCO_2$ > 30 mmHg.	
	Watch for hypoventilation as patient rate ↓. Usually not tolerated well above 300 mL.			

Basic Operating Principles of Volume-Controlled Ventilation

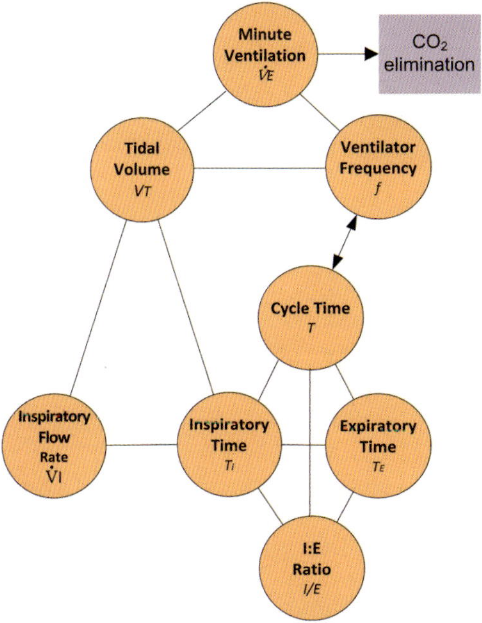

Explanations on next page

Only three parameters are directly adjusted by any one ventilator (this varies with the individual ventilator design). All other factors will be indirectly altered by manipulation of one of those known factors.

Adapted from Chatburn, R.L. and Lough, M.D.: Mechanical Ventilation. In Lough, M.D. et al: ***Pediatric Respiratory Therapy***, copyright 1985 by Mosby Yearbook.

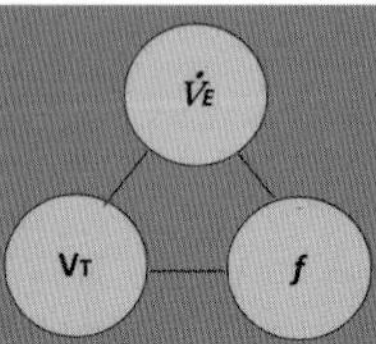

$$\dot{V}_E = V_T \times f$$

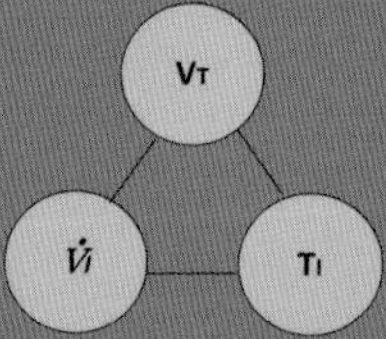

$$V_T = \dot{V}_I \times T_I$$

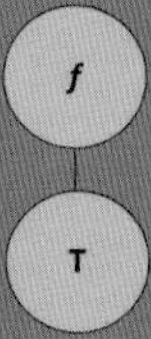

$$T = 60/f$$
$$f = 60/T$$

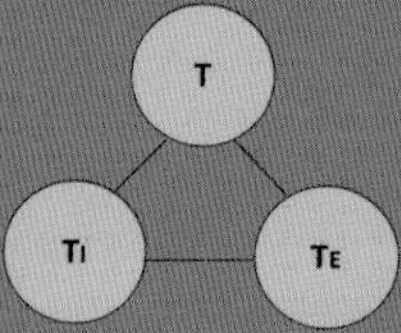

$$T = T_I + T_E$$

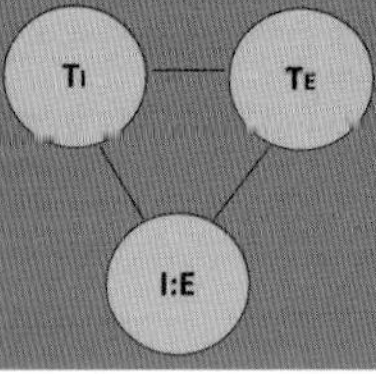

$$I:E = \frac{1}{(T_E/T_I)}$$

Basic Operating Principles of Pressure-Controlled Ventilation

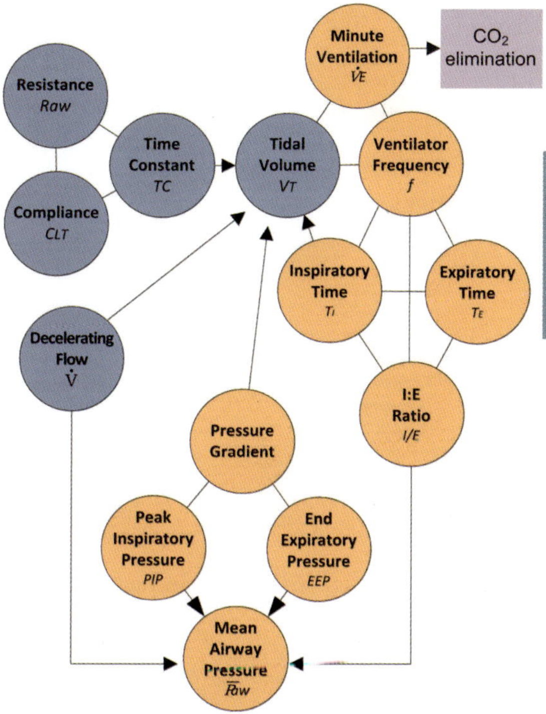

Arrows indicate non-quantifiable, complex relationships.

Orange circles represent variables that are controlled directly by ventilator settings.

Blue circles are controlled indirectly.

Adapted from Chatburn, R.L. and Lough, M.D.: Mechanical Ventilation. In Lough, M.D. et al: ***Pediatric Respiratory Therapy***, copyright 1985 by Mosby Yearbook

Determinants of Oxygenation

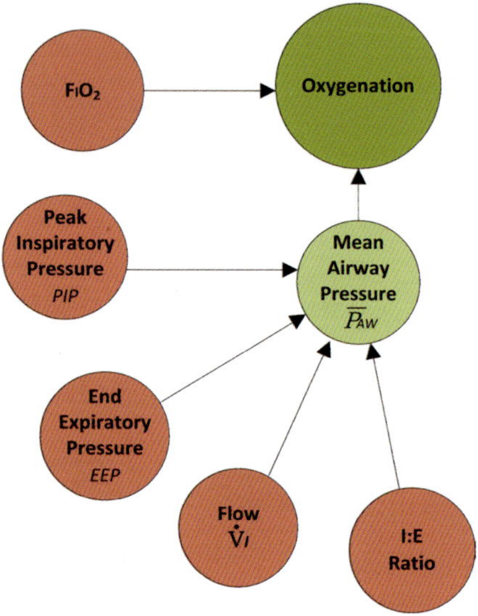

Red circles represent variables that are controlled directly by ventilator settings.

Solid arrows represent the relationships that determine mean airway pressure ($\overline{P}aw$) and oxygenation.

The dashed arrow represents relationships that can't be quantified ($\overline{P}aw$'s impact on oxygenation).

Adapted from Carlo, W.A., Greenough, A. Chatburn, R.L.: Advances in mechanical ventilation. In Boynton B.R., Carlo W.A., Jobe A.H. [Eds.]:***New Therapies for Neonatal Respiratory Failure: A Physiologic Approach***. Cambridge, Cambridge University Press, 1994, p. 134

Notes Page

Make It Your Own

Notes Page

3 Modes of Ventilaton

CONTENTS

MODE CHART 3-2

Each is found by the numerical order on the mode chart

Mode Selection Chart 3-45

Mode Definition: How a ventilator delivers breaths to a patient (breath types *given* or *allowed*).

Mode Classification: A ventilator mode is classified by:

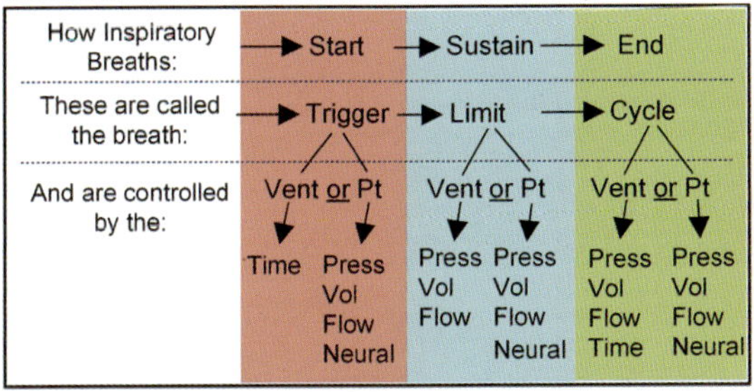

Breath Types

Breaths	Inspiratory Phase Variables		
	Trigger	**Limit**	**Cycle**
Ventilator-Cycled Breaths			
Ventilator (control) breath	MT	ML	MC
Assisted breath	PT	ML	MC
Patient-Cycled breath:			
Supported breath	PT	ML	PC
Spontaneous breath	PT	PL	PC

MT = machine-triggered
ML = machine-limited
MC = machine-cycled

PT = patient-triggered
PL = patient-limited
PC = patient-cycled

Modes of Ventilation[1]

(see mode chart key, page 3-5)

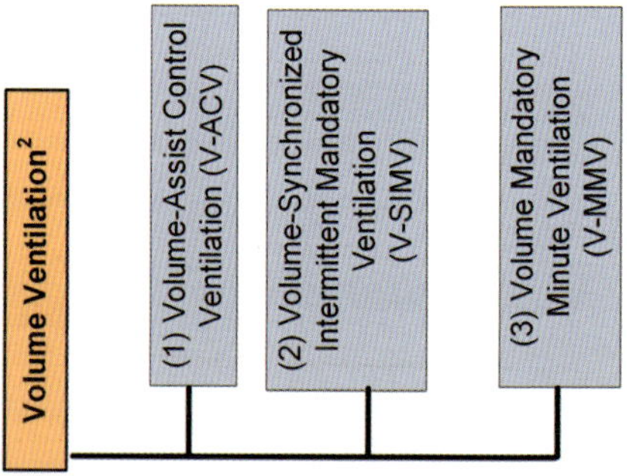

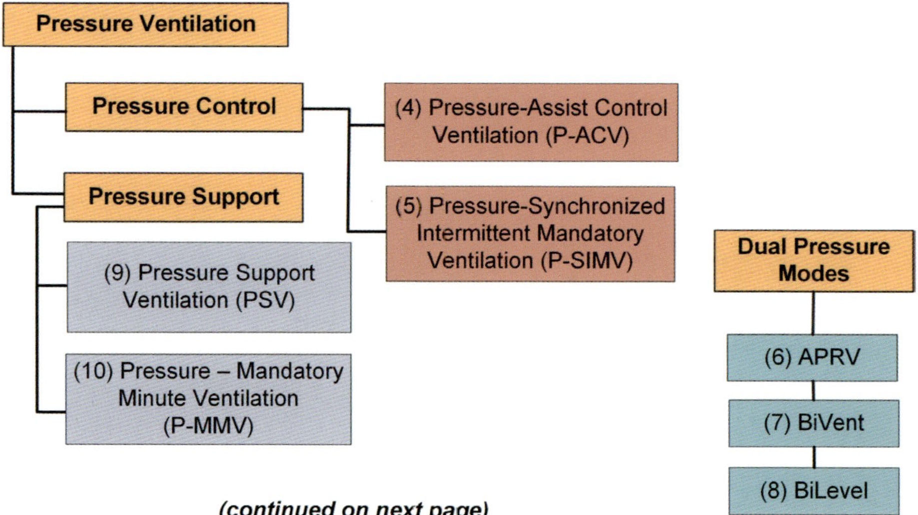

(continued on next page)

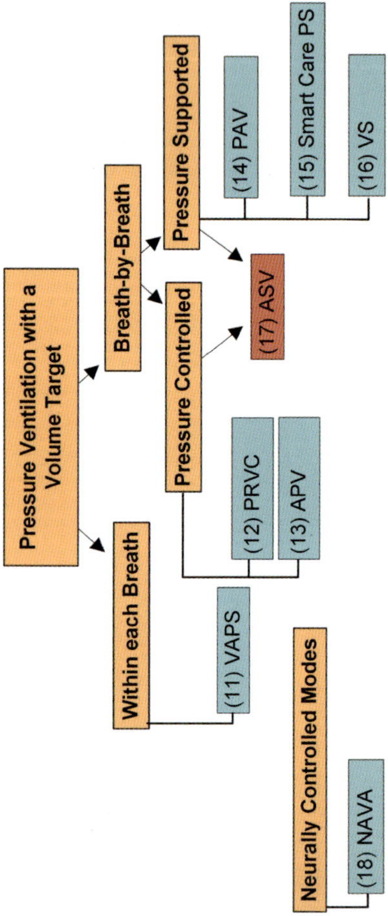
Pressure Ventilation with a Volume Target
Within each Breath
Breath-by-Breath
Pressure Controlled
Pressure Supported
(11) VAPS
(12) PRVC
(13) APV
(14) PAV
(15) Smart Care PS
(16) VS
(17) ASV
Neurally Controlled Modes
(18) NAVA

Mode Key

Use this list with the previous diagrams. Each number is associated with more complete information on the mode in the following pages in this chapter.

Volume Ventilation	
(1) V-ACV	Volume Assist/Control Ventilation
(2) V-SIMV	Volume Synchronized Intermittent Mandatory Ventilation
(3) V-MMV	Volume Mandatory Minute Ventilation
Pressure Ventilation	
(4) P-ACV	Pressure Assist/Control Ventilation
(5) P-SIMV	Pressure Synchronized Intermittent Mandatory Ventilaton
(6) APRV	Airway Pressure Release Ventilation
(7) BiVent	
(8) Bilevel	
(9) PSV	Pressure Support Ventilation
(10) P-MMV	Pressure Mandatory Minute Ventilation
Pressure Ventilation with a Target Volume	
(11) VAPS	Volume Assured Pressure Support
(12) PRVC	Pressure Regulated Volume Control
(13) APV	Adaptive Pressure Ventilation
(14) PAV	Proportional Assist Ventilation
(15) SmartCare PS	Smart Care Pressure Support
(16) VS	Volume Support
(17) ASV	Adaptive Support Ventilation
Neural Control Modes	
(18) NAVA	Neurally Adjusted Ventilatory Assist

Continued Next Page

Other "Modes" (Adjuncts)	
(19) ATC	Automatic Tube Compensation
(20) Automode	Automode
(21) CPAP	Continuous Positive Airway Pressure

1. Modes (names, classifications, etc.) can be very confusing, in part due to manufactuers' reluctance to standardize terminology. What follows in this chapter simplified, quick reference approach to the current modes.
2. Many of these modes lack evidence-based support, making the best choice of mode that which the Therapist/Physician have the most expertise with in the context of the specific patient clinical situation.
3. Volume ventilation can also be called volume-controlled, -cycled, -limited or -targeted ventilation.
4. Flow-limited or flow-controlled is synonymous with volume-limited or volume-controlled.
5. Closed-Loop Ventilation refers to modes that auto-titrate (somehow) in response to changing patient condition. Examples include NAVA, ASV, and Automode (see each for more details)

Initial Settings with Specific Modes:

- The foundational **Initial Settings** for parameters like V_T, PIP, T_I, etc., can be found in detail in Chapter 4.
- **Disease-specific recommendations** (inlcuding mode selection where appropriate) can be found in Chapter 10.
- **Some mode settings** (such as APRV) are beyond the scope of this book, but excellent detailed management information can be found in Oakes' Critical Care Pocket Guide or online at RespiratoryUpdate.com.

1 V-ACV Volume-Assist/Control Ventilation

- A combination of assisted and/or controlled (mandatory) ventilation.
- All breaths are delivered at a set V_T and $\dot{V}_I$
- In between the controlled (set rate) breaths, a patient can trigger a full machine (assisted) breath at the same parameters as the controlled breath (i.e., V_T and $\dot{V}_I$).

Other Names for Volume-Assist/Control

Volume Control
Volume Assist Mechanical Ventilation
Continuous Mechanical Ventilation (CMV)
Assist/Control Volume Control (AC/VC)

Other Names for Assist	Other Names for Control
Assisted Ventilation (AV)	Control Mode
Assisted Mechanical Ventilation (AMV)	Controlled Mechanical Ventilation (CMV)
Volume Assist (VA)	Controlled Mandatory Ventilation (CMV)
Volume Cycled Ventilation (VCV)	Volume Control Ventilation (VCV)
	Volume Cycled Ventilation (VCV)

	Classified By:		
Breath Type	**Trigger**	**Limit**	**Cycle**
Mandatory *(Controlled)*	MT *(Time)*	ML *($\dot{V}$ or Vol)*	MC *(Vol)*
Assisted	PT *(Press or $\dot{V}$)*	ML *($\dot{V}$ or Vol)*	MC *(Vol)*

Indications:

- Patients requiring full ventilatory support. For those who make inadequate or no respiratory effort due to: drugs, cerebral malfunction, spinal cord or phrenic nerve injury, or motor nerve paralysis.
- Used in patients with stable respiratory drives who are able to trigger the ventilator.

Modes

V-ACV

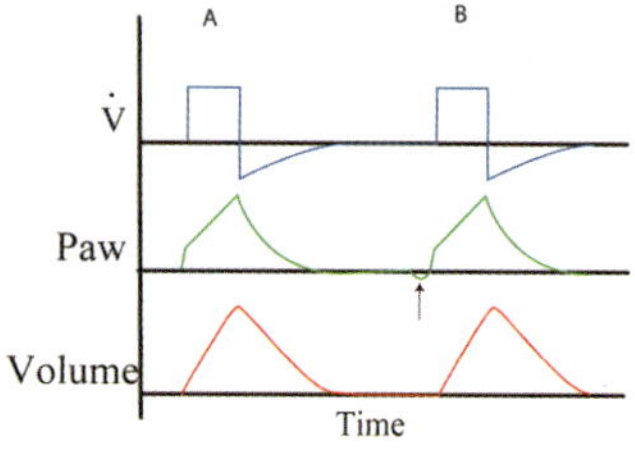

Breath A is Controlled + Machine-Triggered
Breath B is Assisted + Patient-Triggered
Each Breath is a Full Machine-Pressure Breath

Modes

Advantages:

- Maximum ventilatory support
- Guaranteed V_T with a minimum $\dot{V}_E$
- Minimal patient WOB (if parameters are properly adjusted)
- Allows some patient control of *f* and $\dot{V}_E$

Disadvantages:

- High pressure limit must be set appropriately to minimize the risk of alveolar injury
- Excessive patient WOB if flow and sensitivity are not set correctly (asynchrony)
- The flow is fixed, which inhibits the patient who has a ↑ $\dot{V}_I$ or volume demand.
- Possible alveolar hyperventilation and respiratory alkalosis Due to:
  1. Inappropriate sensitivity setting (auto-cycling)
  2. Rapid (assisted) breathing rate
- High risk of cardiovascular compromise
- May be poorly tolerated in awake, nonsedated patients
- May cause or worsen auto-PEEP (dynamic hyperinflation)
- Potential for respiratory muscle atrophy

2	V-SIMV	Volume-Synchronized Intermittent Mandatory Ventilation

A combination of spontaneous and mandatory ventilation.

- The ventilator will deliver a set number of mandatory (controlled) breaths per minute.
- These mandatory breaths will be at a preset V_T and $\dot{V}_I$
- The patient may breathe spontaneously in between the mandatory machine breaths from the baseline pressure. The breath may be assisted with PS.
- If the patient begins to inspire just prior to the time triggered mandatory (control) breath, a full machine-assisted breath will be delivered.

	Classified By:		
Breath Type	**Trigger**	**Limit**	**Cycle**
Mandatory *(Controlled)*	MT *(Time)*	ML *($\dot{V}$ or Vol)*	MC *(Vol)*
Assisted	PT *(Press or $\dot{V}$)*	ML *($\dot{V}$ or Vol)*	MC *(Vol)*
Spontaneous	PT *(Press or $\dot{V}$)*	PL *(Press)*	PC *(Press or $\dot{V}$)*

Modes

Indications:

- Full to partial ventilatory support
- Used after a period of full ventilatory support to transfer respiratory workload back to the patient (See Disadvantages & Risks)

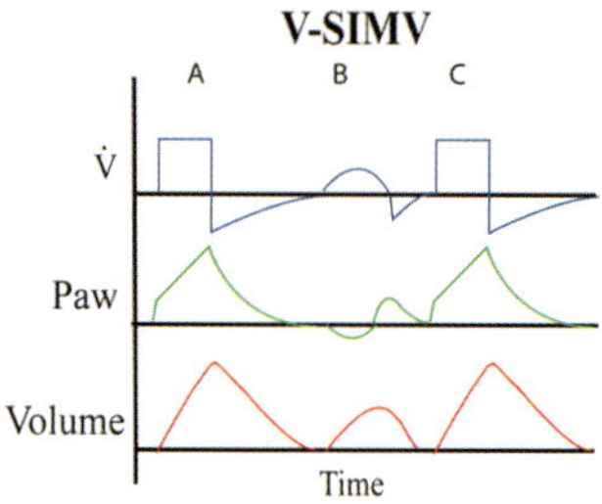

Breath A is Controlled + Time triggered
Breath B is a spontaneous breath (no pressure support)
Breath C is synchronized and assited
Breaths A + C are both full machine volume breaths

Modes

Advantages:

- More tightly controls volume with each mandatory breath.
- Security of a safe minimum $\dot{V}_E$
- May maintain respiratory muscle strength (avoids atrophy)
- Synchronization of spontaneous and mandatory breaths
- Spontaneous breaths may be pressure supported (see PSV)
- Spontaneous breathing generally produces better gas distribution and less Cardiac Output compromise

Disadvantages and Risks:

- High pressure limit must be set appropriately to minimize the risk of alveolar injury
- Patient WOB if flow rate/sensitivity are not set correctly
- Possible tachypnea with fatigue and hypercapnia if mandatory (control) rate is set too low (inadequate ventilatory support or weaning too rapidly)
- ↑ patient WOB for spontaneous breaths unless adequate PSV is added
- Studies suggest that SIMV weaning is associated with the poorest outcomes (longer weaning times). *Hess D. Ventilator modes used in weaning. ***Chest*** 2001; 120:6 Supp. 474S-476S

3	V-MMV	Volume-Mandatory Minute Ventilation

Volume ventilation which guarantees a minimum $\dot{V}_E$. A set minute volume is guaranteed by monitoring the patient's spontaneous minute volume. The ventilator will add supplemental breaths as needed to achieve the set $\dot{V}_E$.

	Classified By:		
Breath Type	**Trigger**	**Limit**	**Cycle**
Mandatory *(Controlled)*	MT *(Time)*	ML *($\dot{V}$ or Vol)*	MC *(Vol)*
Assisted	PT *(Press or $\dot{V}$)*	ML *($\dot{V}$ or Vol)*	MC *(Vol)*
Spontaneous	PT *(Press or $\dot{V}$)*	PL *(Press)*	PC *(Press or $\dot{V}$)*

Other names and abbreviations:

- Minimum Mandatory Ventilation (MMV)
- Augmented Minute Ventilation (AMV)
- Extended Mandatory Minute Ventilation (EMMV)

How it works:

- There is a set $\dot{V}_E$ (this should be thought of as a minimum $\dot{V}_E$)
- If the patient's spontaneous ventilation does not equal or exceed the set $\dot{V}_E$ (VT x *f*), the ventilator rate (RR) is automatically adjusted to meet the minimum set

Indications:

- Patients who are spontaneously breathing or ready to wean
- Patients with unstable ventilatory drive

Advantages:

- Allows spontaneous ventilation with a safety net
- A minimum $\dot{V}_E$ is guaranteed
- Prevents hypoventilation (when V_T is set correctly)

Disadvantages and Risks:

- $\dot{V}_E$ may not equal $\dot{V}_A$ (with rapid shallow breathing)
- The high rate alarm must be set low enough to alert clinician of rapid shallow breathing
- Variable PIP (greater risk of barotrauma)
- An inadequate set $\dot{V}_E$ ($<$ spontaneous $\dot{V}_E$) can lead to inadequate support and patient fatigue
- An excessive set $\dot{V}_E$ ($>$ spontaneous $\dot{V}_E$) with no spontaneous breathing can lead to total support

4	P-ACV	Pressure-Assist/Control Ventilation

- A combination of assisted and/or controlled (mandatory) ventilation
- All breaths are delivered at a preset PIP and T_I
- In between the controlled breaths a patient can trigger a full machine (assisted) breath at the same parameters as the controlled breath (i.e., PIP and T_I)

Caution: Some ventilators (and some versions of the same ventilator) set Pressure Control (PIP) relative to the set PEEP, while in others the set Pressure Control is the "true" PIP (above baseline). Sometimes this is also referred to as **PEEP-compensated** or **not-PEEP-compensated**.

Other Names for Pressure-Assist/Control

Pressure Control
Pressure Assist Mechanical Ventilation

Other Names for Assist	Other Names for Control
Pressure Assist (PA)	Control Mode
Pressure Control Ventilation (PCV)	Controlled Mechanical Ventilation (CMV)
Assisted Ventilation (AV)	Pressure Control Ventilation (PCV)
Assisted Mechanical Ventilation (AMV)	

	Classified By:		
Breath Type	**Trigger**	**Limit**	**Cycle**
Mandatory *(Controlled)*	MT *(Time)*	ML *(Press)*	MC *(Time)*
Assisted	PT *(Press or $\dot{V}$)*	ML *(Press)*	MC *(Time)*

Indications:

- Patients requiring full ventilatory support
  For those who make inadequate or no respiratory effort due to: drugs, cerebral malfunction, spinal cord or phrenic nerve injury, or motor nerve paralysis
- Patients requiring a preset pressure limit and variable inspiratory flow

P-ACV

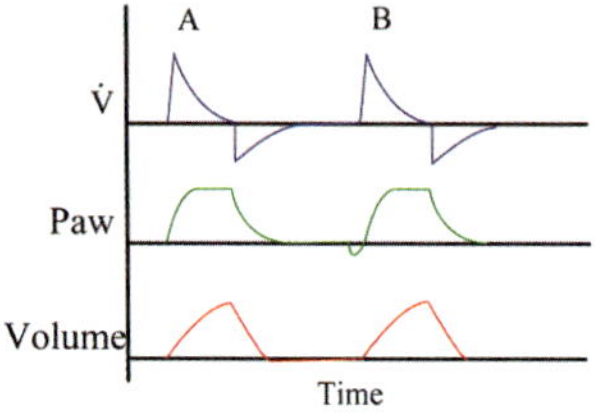

Breath A is controlled and time-triggered
Breath B is assisted and patient-triggered
Each breath is a full machine pressure breath

Advantages:

- Guaranteed pressure limited breaths (minimizes PIP/Pplat)
- Minimal patient WOB (if parameters are properly adjusted)
- Allows patient control of rate and $\dot{V}_E$
- Variable $\dot{V}_I$ may be more comfortable for patients
- Delivers volume early in the breath (decelerating flow) which may improve gas distribution

Disadvantages and Risks:

- No guaranteed V_T (as in volume ventilation)
- Low exhaled V_T and $\dot{V}_E$ alarms must be set properly
- Possible alveolar hyperventilation and possible respiratory alkalosis due to: Inappropriate sensitivity setting (auto-cycling) and/or rapid breathing rate
- Higher risk of cardiovascular compromise
- May cause or worsen auto-PEEP (dynamic hyperinflation)
- Potential respiratory muscle atrophy

5	P-SIMV	Pressure-Synchronized Intermittent Mandatory Ventilation

A combination of spontaneous and mandatory ventilation.

- The ventilator will deliver a set number of mandatory (controlled) breaths per minute
- These mandatory breaths will be at a preset PIP and T_I
- The patient may breathe spontaneously in between the mandatory ventilator breaths from the baseline pressure. The breath may be assisted with PS
- If the patient begins to inspire just prior to the time triggered mandatory (control) breath, a full machine-assisted breath will be delivered

Caution: Some ventilators (and some versions of the same ventilator) have a set Pressure Control (PIP) above the set PEEP, while in others the set Pressure Control is the "true" PIP (above baseline). Sometimes this is also referred to as **PEEP-compensated** or **not-PEEP-compensated**.

	Classified By:		
Breath Type	**Trigger**	**Limit**	**Cycle**
Mandatory *(Controlled)*	MT *(Time)*	ML *(Press)*	MC *(Time)*
Assisted	PT *(Press or $\dot{V}$)*	ML *(Press)*	MC *(Time)*
Spontaneous	PT *(Press or $\dot{V}$)*	PL *(Press)*	PC *(Press or $\dot{V}$)*

Indications:

- Full to partial ventilatory support
- Used after a period of full ventilatory support to begin the transfer of work to the patient (i.e., weaning) (See Disadvantages & Risks)
- Patients requiring a preset PIP and variable $\dot{V}$

Modes

P-SIMV

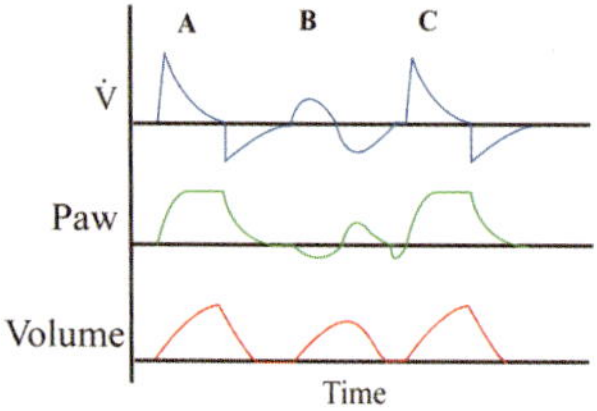

Breath A is controlled and time-triggered
Breath B is a spontaneous breath (no pressure support)
Breath C is synchronized and assisted
Breaths A and C are full machine pressure breaths

Modes

Advantages:

- Guaranteed pressure-limited breaths
- Maintains respiratory muscle strength and minimizes muscle atrophy
- Lowers $\overline{Paw}$
- May reduce respiratory alkalosis associated with A/C
- Synchronization of spontaneous and machine breaths
- Spontaneous breaths may be supported with PS if desirable clinically (See PSV Mode)
- Delivers volume early in the breath, which may improve gas distribution

Disadvantages and Risks:

- No guaranteed V_T. (Set Low V_T and $\dot{V}_E$ alarms carefully)
- Excessive patient WOB if the sensitivity is not set correctly
- Possible tachypnea with fatigue and hypercapnia, if mandatory rate is set too low (i.e., inadequate ventilatory support or weaning too rapidly)
- ↑ patient WOB for spontaneous breaths unless PSV is added
- Studies suggest that SIMV weaning is associated with the poorest outcomes. *Hess D. Ventilator Modes Used in Weaning. ***Chest*** 2001; 120:6 Supp. 474S-476S

6	APRV	Airway Pressure Release Ventilation

Primarily a spontaneous mode of ventilation (spontaneous breaths deliver maximum therapeutic advantage). This mode is basically "inverse ratio" ventilation if patient is not breathing spontaneously

Patient is able to breathe at two Pressure Levels:

1. A longer high level which allows for alveolar recruitment
2. A very short low level (set to therapeutically cause air trapping). The purpose of the low level, also called "the release" is to allow for CO_2 elimination, while maintaining therapeutic air-trapping.

Pressure Support may be added for the spontaneous component of the breath either at the high level (all forms of the mode) and sometimes at the low level (Bi-Vent)

Other names:

- Bilevel (sometimes called BIPAP, but don't confuse this with the Noninvasive form of ventilation called BiPAP).
- Variable Positive Airway Pressure (VPAP)
- Intermittent CPAP
- CPAP with release

	Classified By:		
Breath Type	**Trigger**	**Limit**	**Cycle**
Mandatory *(Controlled)*	MT *(Time)*	ML *(Press)*	MC *(Time)*
Assisted	PT *(Press or $\dot{V}$)*	ML *(Press)*	MC *(Press or $\dot{V}$)*

Ventilator Specific: Drager Evita 2,4,XL; Viasys Avea,Vela; BiLevel-Puritan Bennett 840; Bivent-Maquet Servo I (with BiLevel and Bi-vent, PS breaths can augment spontaneous breaths if the clinician desires), Hamilton Galileo (Duo-PAP)

Note: Each specific ventilator handles spontaneous breaths in its own way. Refer to the manufacturer's manual.

APRV

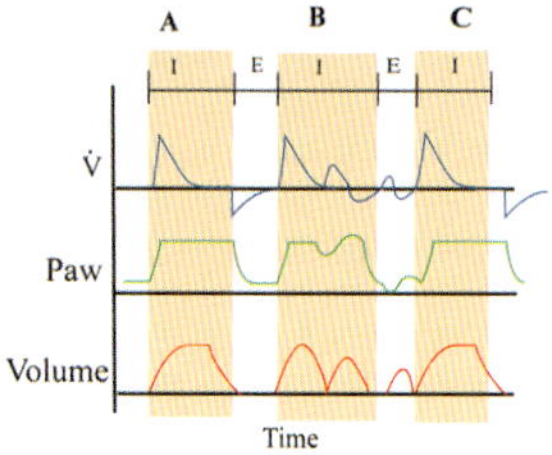

Breath A and C are machine breaths without any spontaneous efforts. Breath B has spontaneous breaths in the I + E phase.

How it works:

- Allows spontaneously breathing patients to breathe at a high CPAP level, and periodically releases - drops briefly - (generally < 1 second) to a low CPAP level for extra CO_2 elimination (airway pressure release)
- Mandatory breaths (Pressure Level) occur when the pressure limit rises from the lower CPAP to the higher CPAP level

Indications:

- May be considered as a mode that prioritizes lung protection (prevention of alveolar trauma)
- Patients with ALI/ARDS
- Patients with refractory hypoxemia due to collapsed alveoli
- Patients with massive atelectasis (recruitment)
- *May use with mild or no lung disease*

Advantages:

- Less sedatives and paralytics required (versus IRV)
- Improves synchrony if spontaneous breathing present.
- Increases/Improves $\overline{Paw}$
- May improve oxygenation by stabilizing collapsed alveoli
- Allows patients to breathe spontaneously while maintaing lung recruitment
- Lowers PIP
- May decrease physiologic deadspace

Disadvantages and Risks:

- Variable V_T
- Could be harmful to patients with high expiratory resistance (i.e., COPD or asthma)
- Auto-PEEP is usually present (by design)
- Caution should be used with hemodynamically unstable patients
- Asynchrony can occur if spontaneous breaths (if present) are out of sync with timed releases
- May not be as familiar to some physicians/critical care nurses
- Requires the presence of an "active exhalation valve"

Modes

7 Bi-Vent

See APRV for technical information on this mode.

Primary difference between this and APRV is that Bi-Vent uses slightly different terminology ($PEEP_{LOW}$ and $PEEP_{HIGH}$), and allows the clinician to set Pressure Support at the low pressure level, not just the high pressure level

8	**Bilevel**
	See APRV for technical information on this mode. *Bilevel, like APRV, has two pressure levels (a high and a low), and the patient may breathe spontaneously during either level.* *Strategy 1: Use conventional I:E ratios or Inverse ratios, but with a longer exhalation time than is typical in APRV.* *Strategy 2: Use the mode similar to how APRV is used, which is inverse ratio with a short exhalation time to cause therapeutic air-trapping.*

How it works:

- The clinician selects a high CPAP level ($PEEP_H$) and a low CPAP level ($PEEP_L$) and a set time for the two levels. This sets the mandatory rate
- The patient may breathe spontaneously at both CPAP levels. These breaths can be pressure supported using the following rules:
  - o Pressure support can assist spontaneous breaths at $PEEP_L$ and $PEEP_H$ (provided there is adequate time at $PEEP_L$)
  - o Pressure support is always relative to PEEP. Target pressure level = $PEEP_L$ + pressure support
  - o Spontaneous breaths at $PEEP_H$ are not supported unless the PS level > ($PEEP_H$-$PEEP_L$). All spontaneous breaths are supported with at least 1.5 cmH_2O
  - o If (pressure support + $PEEP_L$) > ($PEEP_H$ + 1.5 cmH_2O), all of the spontaneous breaths at PEEPL are assisted by PS setting and all spontaneous breaths at $PEEP_H$ are assisted by PS - ($PEEP_H$-$PEEP_L$)
- If the patient does not breathe spontaneously, the mode acts like P-ACV
- The mandatory breaths occur when the pressure limit rises from the lower PEEP level to the higher PEEP level

See APRV for complete Technical Description, Indications, Advantages and Disadvantages and Risks

Modes

9	PSV	Pressure Support Ventilation
	Spontaneous ventilation with all of the patient's spontaneous breaths supported or augmented by the ventilator (a set pressure is added to each spontaneous breath)	

Other names:

- Inspiratory Assist (IA)
- Inspiratory Pressure Support (IPS)
- Spontaneous Pressure Support (SPS)
- Inspiratory Flow Assist (IFA)

	Classified By:		
Breath Type	**Trigger**	**Limit**	**Cycle**
Supported	PT *(Press or $\dot{V}$)*	PL *(Press)*	PC *($\dot{V}_I$)**

*Pressure Supported breaths are generally flow cycled (as inspiratory flow slows, the ventilator reads this as the patient being ready to start exhalation), but may be pressure-cycled or time-cycled as a back-up measure on some ventilators

Modes

How it works:

- A pressure support level is set by the clinician, usually not less than 10 cmH_2O. This may be titrated to a desired V_T, but the clinician should remain aware that because pressure is set, V_T will vary with changes in compliance, resistance, and patient effort
- Inspiratory phase ends when the inspiratory flow rate reaches a set minimum flow rate or percentage of the patient's peak flow (ventilator specific). Some newer ventilators have variable cycling criteria known as "expiratory sensitivity" and "inspiratory cycle off". There are also pressure and time cycling criteria as back up measures available on some ventilators.

Indications:

- Spontaneously breathing patients who require additional ventilatory support to help overcome:
  ↑ WOB (↓ C or ↑ Raw) or respiratory muscle weakness
- Weaning

PSV

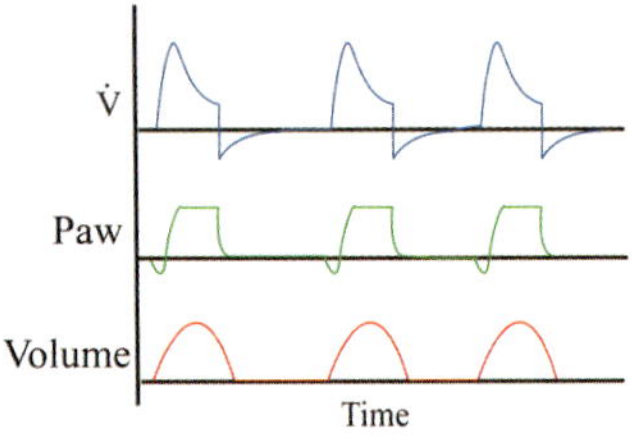

Advantages:

- Supports the patient's spontaneous V_T
- MAY decrease the patient's spontaneous RR
- MAY decrease patient WOB by overcoming the resistance of the artificial airway, vent circuit and demand valves.
- Allows greater patient control of T_I, $\dot{V}_I$, *f* and V_T
- Improves patient comfort and reduces need for sedation
- May be applied in any mode that allows spontaneous breath
- Minimizes respiratory muscle atrophy
- Lowers $\overline{P}aw$
- Facilitates weaning

Modes

Disadvantages and Risks:

- Requires consistent spontaneous ventilation (back-up ventilation and appropriate alarms must be ensured)
- V_T variable and dependent on lung characteristics and synchrony
- The expiratory cycling criteria vary depending on the ventilator used. Cycling asynchrony could occur
- Fatigue and tachypnea if PS level is set too low (If patient using sternocleidomastoid muscles consider ↑ the PS level)
- Auto-PEEP if PS level is set too high (If the PS level is decreased and there is no change in the V_T or accessory muscle use, consider leaving at the new level)

10	P-MMV	Pressure-Mandatory Minute Ventilation
	Spontaneous mode of ventilation with a variable pressure support (pressure added to each spontaneous breath). This support titrates to maintain a minimum set $\dot{V}_E$	

Other names and abbreviations:

- Minimum Mandatory Ventilation (MMV)
- Augmented Minute Ventilation (AMV)
- Extended Mandatory Minute Ventilation (EMMV)

How it works:

- If the patient's spontaneous ventilation does not equal or exceed the set $\dot{V}_E$ (V_T x f), the ventilator delivers the difference between the actual and set target $\dot{V}_E$
- The difference is provided by the ventilator changing the PS of the spontaneous breaths
- If the patient exceeds the set $\dot{V}_E$, no ventilator support is added

Indications:

- Any patient who is spontaneously breathing and is deemed ready to wean
- Patients with unstable ventilatory drive

Advantages:

- Allows spontaneous ventilation with a safety net
- Prevents hypoventilation ($\dot{V}_E$ remains relatively stable)

Disadvantages and Risks:

- An adequate $\dot{V}_E$ may not equal sufficient $\dot{V}_A$ (e.g., rapid shallow breathing)
- The high rate alarm must be set low enough to alert clinician of rapid shallow breathing
- Variable $\bar{P}aw$
- An inadequate set $\dot{V}_E$ (< spontaneous $\dot{V}_E$) can lead to inadequate support and patient fatigue
- An excessive set $\dot{V}_E$ (> spontaneous $\dot{V}_E$) with no spontaneous breathing can lead to total support

11	VAPS	Volume-Assured Pressure Support

Breaths start out as Pressure Supported (pressure added to each spontaneous breath), but as inspiratory flow begins to decrease, the ventilator checks the delivered volume against a Target V_T that the clinician has set. If the volume is adequate, the ventilator cycles into exhalation. If the volume is too low, the ventilator maintains flow until that set volume has been delivered.

May be used with A/C, SIMV, or CPAP (during Apnea)

Other names: Volume-Assisted Pressure Support

Variation: Pressure Augmentation (P_{aug}): patient must be able to intiate a breath and have a consistent RR

	Classified By:		
Breath Type	**Trigger**	**Limit**	**Cycle**
Mandatory ***(Controlled)***	MT *(Time)*	PL *(Press or Vol)*	PC *(Vol or $\dot{V}$)*
Assisted	PT *(Press or $\dot{V}$)*	PL *(Press or $\dot{V}$)*	PC *(Vol or $\dot{V}$)*
Supported	PT *(Press or $\dot{V}$)*	PL *(Press)*	PC *($\dot{V}$)*

Indications:

- Spontaneous breathing patients who require minimum V_T
- Patients who are asynchronous with the ventilator
- Used as a back-up safety net for pressure support ventilation (to ensure a minimum V_T for each breath)

Advantages:

- Volume guaranteed with each breath
- High variable flow for improved synchrony
- Pressure-limited breath for improved gas mixing/oxygenation *
- Decreased patient WOB

* When the ventilator switches to a volume ventilation breath, the pressure limiting advantage is lost

VAPS

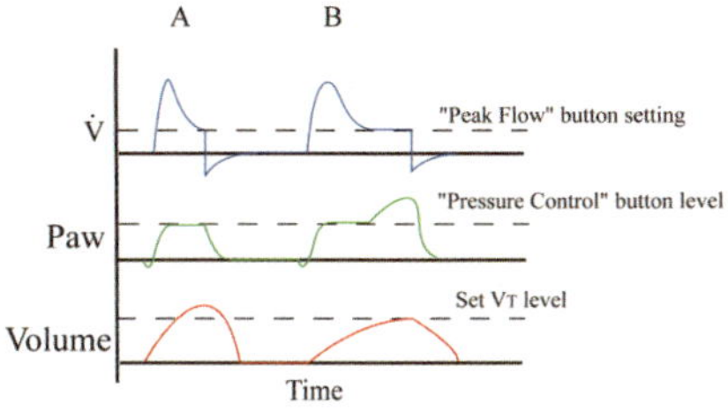

Breath A: Depicts a PS-like breath that has been terminated at the set "Peak Flow" after the minimum V_T has been delivered.

Breath B: Depicts a transition from a PS-like breath to a volume assured (controlled) breath. Transition occurs when flow has decelerated to the set "Peak Flow" and the set V_T has not been delivered. The I-time is extended until the set V_T is delivered.

How it works:

- When a VAPS breath is delivered, the breath is delivered using whatever pressure level is set ("Pressure Control" button on the front panel).
- If the set minimum V_T is achieved by the time the flow ↓ to the set flow-cycle value ("Peak Flow" button on the front panel), the ventilator cycles into exhalation. In this case, the breath acts as a normal PS breath. The V_T could be exceeded.
- If the set V_T is not achieved, the flow is maintained as a constant flow pattern at the set "peak flow" value until the set V_T is achieved. The breath then acts as a volume-cycled breath.
- If the breath becomes a volume-cycled breath, the resulting pressure will be higher than the set pressure support level

Note: Determining the correct pressure level is complex and no studies have been done to show the best settings.

Disadvantages and Risks:

- Choosing the appropriate pressure and flow settings are crucial for successful and safe operation. *Examples*:
  - If the "peak flow" (flow-cycle value) is set too high, all the breaths will switch from pressure to volume-cycled, which will defeat the purpose of using the mode
  - If the "peak flow" is set too low, the inspiratory time could be too long to achieve the desired set V_T and I:E
  - If the pressure is set too high, the volume back-up will never be needed
  - If the pressure is set too low and/or the V_T is set too low, the patient could become distressed and/or under-ventilated
- Varying $\overline{P}aw$
- A sudden ↑ in RR and demand may result in a ↓ in ventilator support

Modes

12	PRVC	Pressure-Regulated Volume Control
	This is, at its foundation, a pressure controlled mode, but adds a target tidal volume, so that the inspiratory pressure changes breath-by-breath up to a set point in order to maintain a stable VT	

Ventilator Specific: PRVC-Maquet Servo I; Servo 300/300A **Viasys Avea and Viasys Vela

Other Names: Variable Pressure Control (VPC),
Volume Control Plus (VCP, VC+)
**Refer to the manufacturer's manual (algorithms slightly different)

	Classified By:		
Breath Type	**Trigger**	**Limit**	**Cycle**
Mandatory	MT *(Time)*	ML *(Press or Vol)*	MC *(Time)*
Assisted	PT *(Press or $\dot{V}$)*	ML *(Press or Vol)*	MC *(Time)*

How it works:

- For the first breath, the ventilator gives a volume breath with a pause (plateau)
- The second breath will be a pressure breath at that plateau pressure from the previous breath
- The ventilator will then titrate the inspiratory pressure by no more than 3 cmH_2O from one breath to the next in order to try to meet the target V_T
- As a safety, the maximum available pressure level is 5 cmH_2O below the preset upper pressure alarm (alarm will sound at this point and the breath will switch into exhalation, meaning the set V_T will not be fully delivered - the ventilator will only deliver the amount of volume that it can before hitting that upper limit)
- The minimum inspiratory pressure limit is the baseline setting (PEEP)
- The patient will receive a minimum number of time-triggered mandatory breaths per minute (as in P-ACV)
- PRVC can be combined with SIMV (PRVC-SIMV) so that mandatory breaths are PRVC breaths, and spontaneous are PSV breaths

PRVC

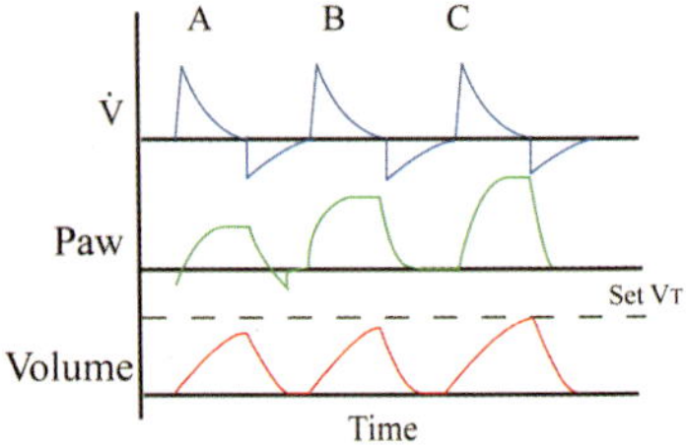

As the breaths advance from A to C, the pressure is automatically increased to achieve the set V_T.

Modes

Indications:
Indications are similar to Pressure A/C

Advantages:

- Guaranteed V_T and $\dot{V}_E$
- Patient can breathe above the set *f*
- Allows patient control of RR and $\dot{V}_E$
- Variable $\dot{V}_I$ (decelerating) to meet patient demand and improve gas distribution

Disadvantages and Risks:

- **Upper pressure limit (alarm) must be set appropriately**
- Excessive patient work of breathing if sensitivity is not set correctly
- May cause or worsen auto-PEEP
- Patients who assist the ventilator by taking larger V_T will cause the inspiratory pressure to drop (as the ventilator drops it in increments of 3's to try to get to goal V_T). If the patient then tires, the ventilator could be delivering as low as the PEEP level at a time when the patient most needs the support. A PIP dropping to PEEP level is a warning of this likelihood.

13	APV	Adaptive Pressure Ventilation
	This mode is nearly identical to PRVC. Differences include: pressure is titrated in 1 cmH_2O increments (versus 3 cmH_2O in PRVC); maximum pressure is 10 cmH_2O below high Pressure alarm (versus 5 cmH_2O), and low pressure is 5 cmH_2O above set PEEP (versus 0 cmH_2O).	

Ventilator Specific: Hamilton Galileo, Hamilton G5

How it works:

- The ventilator continuously calculates system and patient Compliance, and volume delivery
- If the exhaled V_T is less or more than the set V_T, the inspiratory pressure level is regulated until the preset volumes are delivered. Pressure changes are made in 1 cmH_2O increments
- Maximum available inspiratory pressure level is 10 cmH_2O below the set upper pressure limit
- The amount of pressure cannot be set lower than 5 cmH_2O above the baseline pressure (PEEP)
- The patient will receive a minimum number of time-triggered mandatory breaths per minute. (Set back-up rate)

Indications:

Indications are similar to Pressure A/C

Advantages:

- May be used with any Volume mode (V-ACV, V-SIMV, and V-MMV), but changes volume to pressure with volume target
- The expiratory valve is floating, which allows the patient to cough or breathe during the inspiratory time of the mandatory breath while maintaining the achieved inspiratory pressure without a significant under- or overshoot

Disadvantages and Risks:

- Upper pressure limit must be set appropriately (start with 5-10 cmH_2O above Pplat, then adjust as necessary)

14	PAV	Proportional Assist Ventilation
	Mode delivers flow, volume, and pressure based upon the patient's needs (as determined by patient effort), at a percentage set by the clinician. The goal is to standardize the patient's WOB.	

Ventilator Specific: Drager Evita 4 and XL, Puritan Bennett 840 (PAV+)

**Refer to manufacturer's manual

Other names: Proportional Pressure Support (PPS), PAV +

Technical Description:

- Patient-triggered breaths that are provided proportionately to the patient during inspiration
- Incorporates both a "flow assist" and a "volume assist" in proportion to patient demand
- The greater the patient effort, the higher the flow, volume, and pressure

Modes

	Classified By:		
Breath Type	**Trigger**	**Limit**	**Cycle**
Assisted	PT *(Press or $\dot{V}$)*	ML *(Press)*	MC *($\dot{V}$)*

How it works:

- Set the ventilator's volume and flow assist at approximately 80% of the patient's elastance and resistance (↓ as the condition improves)
- The modes works with **assisted breaths only**
- The ventilator then senses the patient's effort to breathe (flow and volume)
- The ventilator then generates proportional flow and volume assist pressures to augment the patient's own effort
- The greater the patient effort, the greater the pressures the machine generates
- The delivered volume or pressure then varies according to the patient's inspiratory effort. (The % of the patient WOB [20%] remains the same regardless of changes in C or Raw)
- Determination of pattern of breathing is shifted to the patient

PAV

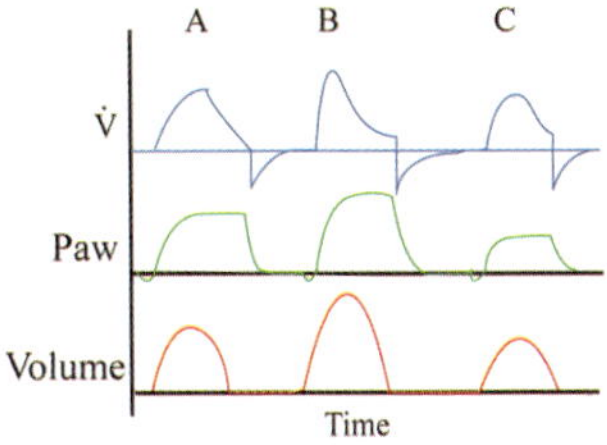

The effort and pressure are increased in Breath B compared to Breath A. The effort and pressure are decreased in Breath C.

Indications:

- Pts who have WOB problems with worsening lung characteristics
- Asynchronous patients who are stable with an inspiratory effort
- Ventilator-dependent patients with COPD

Advantages:

- The patient controls the ventilatory variables ($\dot{V}_I$, PIP, T_I, T_E, V_T)
- Trends the changes of ventilatory effort over time
- When used with CPAP, inspiratory muscle work is near that of a normal subject and may decrease or prevent muscle atrophy
- Lowers airway pressures

Disadvantages and Risks:

- Patient must have adequate spontaneous respiratory drive
- Variable V_T and/or PIP
- Excessive assist ("Runaway") by the ventilator may occur (High V_T and pressure alarms must be set appropriately)
- Air leak could cause excessive assist or automatic cycling
- Trigger effort may increase with auto-PEEP
- Backup mode required in case of apnea
- Correct determination of C and Raw is essential, yet difficult. Both under and over estimates of C and Raw (or changes in C and Raw, as with repositioning) may significantly impair proper patient-ventilator interaction

15	SmartCare PS	Smart Care Pressure Support
	An automated weaning technique that automatically adjusts pressure support levels, to comfortably maintain a patient's breathing frequency, tidal volume and end-tidal CO_2 parameters within predetermined ranges	

Ventilator Specific: Drager Evita XL (optional)

How It Works:

- There are 3 sets of values based on actual body weight
- Each body weight range (15-35 kg, 26-55 kg, and over 55 kg) has different criteria for acceptable tidal volume and frequency
- Based on the patient's initial frequency, tidal volume and $etCO_2$, Smartcare assigns the patient's ventilation to one of eight categories: normal ventilation, insufficient ventilation, hypoventilation, central hypoventilation, tachypnea, severe tachypnea, hyperventilation, or unexplained hyperventilation.
- The clinician also may select "COPD" or "Neurological Disorder" to allow different acceptable parameters (eg., higher $P_{ET}CO_2$)
- Ventilation other than normal will increase or decrease PS by 2-4 cmH_2O (based upon which parameter is out-of-range)
- Smartcare assesses the patient's RR, V_T and $etCO_2$ every 10 seconds and analyzes ventilation every two minutes if there was no PS change or every 5 minutes if there was a PS change
- When the target pressure is obtained, a spontaneous breathing test is performed and if predetermined weight-based values are met a message "SC-Consider Separation" is displayed suggesting to the clinician that liberation may be possible

Indications:

- Spontaneously breathing patients weighing 15-200 kg
- Patients who are screened for the ventilator weaning process

Advantages:

- Ability to have patient frequently assessed mechanically.
- Possibly improved weaning times

Disadvantages and Risks:

- Clinician must still use bedside assessment and judgment
- $EtCO_2$ results will be off if any V/Q mismatch present

16	VS	Volume Support
	This mode could be viewed as "PRVC for spontaneous breathing" as it delivers a variable pressure to meet a target V_T	

Other Names: Volume Support + (Puritan Bennett)
Ventilator Specific: Maquet Servo I

** Volume Support algorithm will be different for the Servo 300A ventilator (VS on the Servo 300/300A is $\dot{V}_E$ based).

	Classified By:		
Breath Type	**Trigger**	**Limit**	**Cycle**
Supported	PT *(Press or $\dot{V}$)*	PL *(Press or Vol)*	PC *($\dot{V}$ or Time)*

Modes

How it works:

- The ventilator gives a test breath with an inspiratory pressure of 10 cmH_2O above PEEP (5 cmH_2O in earlier software versions)
- It measures the volume delivered and calculates system Compliance
- For each subsequent breath, the ventilator calculates compliance of the previous breath and adjusts the inspiratory pressure level (pressure support) to achieve the set V_T on the next breath
- The ventilator will not change the inspiratory pressure more than 3 cmH_2O from one breath to the next
- Maximum available inspiratory pressure level is 5 cmH_2O below the preset upper pressure limit (alarm will sound at this point and the breath will switch into exhalation)
- The minimum pressure limit is the baseline setting (PEEP)
- If apnea occurs, back up pressure support is activated and an alarm sounds
- If Automode is on and patient becomes apneic, the mode will automatically switch to PRVC (See Automode)

VS

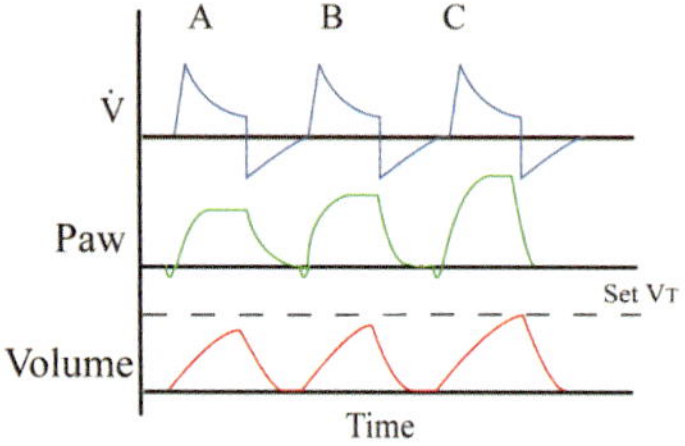

In this example, as the breaths advance from A to C, the pressure is automatically increased to achieve the set V_T. All breaths are patient-triggered breaths.

Modes

Indications:

- Spontaneous breathing patients who require minimum V_T
- Patients who have inspiratory efforts who need added support
- Patients who are asynchronous with the ventilator
- Used for patients who are ready to wean

Advantages:

- Guaranteed V_T and $\dot{V}_E$
- Pressure supported breaths using the lowest required pressure
- Decreases the patient's spontaneous RR and WOB
- Allows patient control of Inspiratory and Expiratory Times (and I:E ratio)
- Variable $\dot{V}_I$ to meet the patient's demand

Disadvantages and Risks:

- Spontaneous ventilation required
- Variable $\overline{P}aw$
- Auto-PEEP may affect operation
- Patients who assist the ventilator by taking larger VT will cause the inspiratory pressure to drop (as the ventilator drops it in increments of 3's to try to get to goal VT). If the patient then tires, the ventilator could be delivering as low as the PEEP level at a time when the patient most needs the support. A PIP dropping to PEEP level is a warning of this likelihood.

17	ASV	Adaptive Support Ventilation
	A dual control mode that uses Pressure Ventilation (both Pressure Control and Pressure Support) to maintain a set minimum $\dot{V}_E$ (volume target) using the least required settings for minimal WOB depending on the patient's condition and effort	

Other Names: Adaptive Tidal Volume Support (AVtS) (same mode except there is greater clinician control over set values)

Ventilator Specific: Hamilton Galileo, G5

	Classified By:		
Breath Type	**Trigger**	**Limit**	**Cycle**
Mandatory	MT *(Time)*	MI *(Press)*	MC *(Time)*
Supported	PT *(Press or $\dot{V}$)*	PL *(Press)*	PC *($\dot{V}$, P, Time)*

How It Works:

- The clinician enters the patient's IBW, which allows the ventilator's algorithm to choose a required $\dot{V}_E$
- The ventilator delivers 100 mL/min/kg
- The clinician can alter the algorithm by adjusting from 20% - 200% the amount of minute ventilation guaranteed (so this will increase ventilator - Pressure Control - contribution if patient does not meet it with spontaneous - Pressure Supported - effort)
- Test breaths measure the system C, resistance, and auto-PEEP
- With no spontaneous breaths, the algorithm adjusts to a *f*, V_T, and pressure limit delivered for the mandatory breaths
- The I:E ratio and T_I of the mandatory breaths are continuously being "optimized" by the ventilator to prevent auto-PEEP
- As the patient initiates, the number of mandatory breaths ↓ and the ventilator switches to PS at the same pressure level
- The spontaneous and mandatory breaths are combined to meet the $\dot{V}_E$ target
- More spontaneous (PS) breathing = less mandatory (PC) breaths
- The ventilator also calculates the expiratory time constant and adjusts the I:E of mandatory breaths to minimize auto-PEEP

Modes

Indications:

- Full or partial ventilatory support
- Patients requiring a lowest possible PIP and a guaranteed V_T
- ARDS (mild-severe)
- Patients requiring high and/or variable $\dot{V}$
- Patients not breathing spontaneously and not triggering the ventilator
- Patients with the possibility of work load changes (C and Raw)
- Facilitates weaning

Advantages:

- Guaranteed V_T and $\dot{V}_E$
- Minimizes patient WOB
- Ventilator adapts to the patient
- Weaning is done automatically and continuously
- Variable $\dot{V}$ to meet patient demand
- Decelerating flow waveform for improved gas distribution
- Breath by breath analysis

Modes

Disadvantages and Risks:

- Inability to recognize and adjust to Δ in alveolar V_D
- Potential respiratory atrophy
- Variable $\overline{P}aw$
- In patients with COPD, a longer T_E may be required
- A sudden ↑ in RR and demand may result in a ↓ in ventilator support.

18	NAVA	Neurally Adjusted Ventilatory Assist

This noninvasive or invasive mode incorporates neural triggering (through a sensor on a specialized NG catheter - positioned in the esophagus near the diaphragm) with spontaneous breaths that are pressure supported proportionally to the strength of the electrical signal from the diaphragm.

Ventilator Specific: Maquet Servo I (optional)

Breath Type		Classified By: Trigger	Limit	Cycle
NAVA	Spontaneous	PT *(Neurally, Press or $\dot{V}$)*	PL *(Neurally)*	PC *(Neurally)*
NAVA (PS)	Spontaneous	PT *(Press or $\dot{V}$)*	PL *(Press)*	PC *($\dot{V}$, P, Time)*
NAVA BACKUP	Mandatory	MT *(Time)*	ML *(Press)*	MC *(Time)*
NAVA BACKUP	Assisted	PT *(Press or Vol)*	ML *(Press)*	MC *(Time)*

How It Works:

- A special functioning Nasogastric tube with an array of measuring electrodes (Edi catheter) is positioned in the esophagus so that the set of measuring electrodes span the path of movement of the diaphragm.
- A calculation based on physical landmarks and the Edi positioning screen assist the clinician on the proper placement of the Edi catheter
- The ventilator receives signals from the Edi catheter and uses those signals for ventilatory monitoring and regulation
- The clinician can set the level of support proportional to the Edi.
- Inspiration is triggered by activation of the Edi signal (neurally), but may also be triggered by Pressure or Flow
- Back-up systems include a back up pressure support if the

neural respiratory rate and timing differs from the pneumatic rate and time. This may be caused by an Edi catheter that has moved. The clinician sets a backup PS level with a trigger and cycle off criteria.

- If case of an apnea (resulting in a permanently low Edi signal and no pneumatic trigger), the ventilator will switch to NAVA backup (pressure control) after the adjustable apnea limit is reached

Indications:

- Mode is used in neonatal - adult populations
- NAVA monitoring (Edi) alone may be done on any patient in any mode of ventilation
- Spontaneously breathing patients
- Patients who are dys-synchronous on conventional modes of ventilation

Advantages:

- Reduced work of breathing—less missed patient trigger efforts. Intrinsic PEEP will not affect triggering in NAVA
- Improved synchrony—the patient's neural and diaphragmatic electrical activity control onset, breath delivery and cycling off of the breath. Synchrony with the ventilator is an important part of unloading the work of the diaphragm, during both inspiration and expiration
- Reduced need for sedation/paralysis – by allowing the patient to control his breathing pattern, less sedation may be required
- Improvement in ventilation, compared to standard methods, by allowing neural triggering, cycling and neurally-adjusted ventilator assistance (e.g., patients with severe airflow impairment)

Disadvantages and Risks:

- The validity of the Edi data (electrical activity) is based upon correct placement of the NG catheter. Any displacement will interfere with the mode (a back-up system as outlined above is in place)
- Can not be used if the respiratory center, phrenic nerve and neuromuscular junction are not intact
- The Edi signal may not be present if patient is over ventilated. This may be a result of too high of a pressure support level or NAVA level if in NAVA mode

19	ATC	Automatic Tube Compensation
	This is an adjunct, but significant enough to be considered in modes. The goal is to overcome WOB created by the artificial airway. It does this by giving variable pressure support (more during inspiration than exhalation) which is proportional to the inspiratory flow and the Internal Diameter (input by the clinician) of the ET Tube.	

Ventilator Specific: Drager Evita 4 and XL and PB 840 (Tube Compensation), Viasys Avea and Hamilton Galileo

How it works:

- The clinician enters ET tube size (ID). The ventilator monitors patient's inspiratory flow.
- The airway pressure (PS) is ↑ during I and ↓ during E to overcome the resistance (the expiratory portion can be disabled)
- The pressure assists in expiration of mandatory breaths and both phases of all spontaneous breaths
- The pressure can be as high as 5 cmH_2O below the upper pressure limit and as low as 0 cmH_2O.
- The clinician sets the % of compensation desired (1%-100%)

Indications:

- Any mechanically ventilated patient with an artificial airway

Advantages:

- Goal is just to overcome resistance of artificial airway, separate from support patient needs
- Superior to PSV for compensation of resistance of artificial airway (i.e., ↓WOB and ↑patient comfort)
- Supports expiration as well as inspiration if desired

Disadvantages and Risks:

- Incomplete compensation may occur with kinks or bends in the artificial airway and secretions in the inner lumen
- In patients with COPD, small airways may be kept open by PEEP and ETT resistance; therefore ATC may need to be inactive for the expiratory portion
- Adding ATC to another mode may result in over assist, in which

case, the primary support level may need to be reduced. This needs to be particularly noted during weaning attempts (SBT) using Pressure Support as the patient is potentially receiving more PS than what is "dialed in" to the ventilator (ATC adds variable PS to the already set PS)

20	Automode	Automode
	Automode, when activated, switches between a more controlled mode (PRVC, P-A/C, V-A/C) and a spontaneous mode (PS, VS). When the patient is triggering the ventilator they are able to breathe on the support side; when they are apneic they will breathe on the control side.	

Ventilator Specific: Maquet Servo 300A, Servo I

How it works:

- While in a control mode, if the patient has two consecutive triggering efforts, the ventilator will switch to a support mode. If the patient becomes apneic*, the ventilator will switch back to the control mode

*Apnea times with Automode only (300A)

Adult	12 seconds
Pediatric	8 seconds
Neonatal	5 seconds

(Apnea times are clinician set with the Servo I by setting "Trigger Timeout")

Control modes partner with support modes as follows:

Control Mode	⟷	Support Mode
Volume Control	⟷	Volume Support
Pressure Control	⟷	Pressure Support
Pressure Reg. Volume Control	⟷	Volume Support

- If switching to VS, the ventilator uses the following formula to determine the inspiratory pressure:
  Set P = {(PIP-PEEP) x 0.5 + PEEP}

See the following Modes for complete descriptions:

- Volume Control on Maquet 300A and Servo I is V-A/C
- Pressure Control on Maquet 300A and Servo I is P-A/C
- Pressure Regulated Volume Support
- Volume Support

Indications:

- Allows ventilator to adapt to the patient's breathing efforts
- Used to facilitate weaning (discontinuation)

See indications for the separate control and support modes.

Advantages:

- Shifts work to patient when ventilator detects two consecutive patient efforts (one breath with the Servo Inspiration)
- Shifts the work to ventilator if patient becomes apneic

See advantages for the separate control and support modes

Disadvantages and Risks:

- Possibility of ↑ WOB
- No alarm is activated when shift occurs (visual signal only)
- Should not be used in patients with neuromuscular blockade or other drug that severely depresses the respiratory drive.
- Switching from time-cycled to flow cycle ventilation may drop $\overline{P}aw$
- Settings must be set appropriately for both the control and support mode being utilized
- Trigger sensitivity must be set appropriately. Auto-triggering would be sensed as patient-triggered breaths, causing it to switch to the support mode

See disadvantages and risks for the separate control and support modes.

21	CPAP	Continuous Positive Airway Pressure
	Spontaneous mode with a constant pressure being held during inspiration and exhalation (similar to having a patient on just PEEP and FIO_2 with no other variables)	

Intubated patients only (See NPPV Chapter for CPAP noninvasively)

Other names:

- Continuous Distending Pressure (CDP)
- Continuous Positive Pressure Breathing (CPPB)

	Classified By:		
Breath Type	**Trigger**	**Limit**	**Cycle**
Spontaneous	PT *(Press or $\dot{V}$)*	PL *(Press)*	PC *(Press or $\dot{V}$)*

Indications:

- Generally indicated for use in spontaneous breathing trials (SBT) during the discontinuation (weaning) process

Advantages:

- Increases FRC while patient remains intubated
- Improves oxygenation if hypoxemia is due to ↓ lung volume
- It may recruit collapsed lung units and minimize the WOB
- It may reduce WOB in patients with dynamic hyperinflation and auto-PEEP

Disadvantages and Risks:

- **No ventilatory support** (patients must support own $\dot{V}_E$)
- Low exhaled $\dot{V}_E$ (low exhaled V_T and high respiratory rate) may go undetected if alarms are not set properly)
- May ↑ WOB if patient unable to maintain adequate $\dot{V}_E$
- Hyperinflation and ↑ expiratory work may result if excessive levels are used
- Does not compensate for resistance of artificial airway

Modes

CPAP

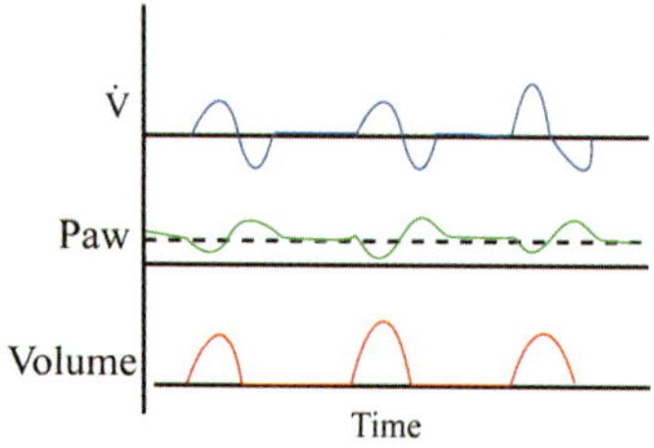

Mode Selection Chart

The following are suggestions for utilizing modes. Obviously this should not take the place of good critical thinking and is not universal!

Full Support	• Assist-Control (A/C) Modes • MMV • PRVC or APV-cmv
Oxygen-ation	• APRV • Bi-Vent • IRV (with caution)
Lung Protective	• APRV • Bi-Vent • HFOV • "Conventional" Modes (A/C) with low V_T strategies
Asynchrony	• NAVA • VAPS • PSV • VSV / ASV
Weaning Modes	• PSV • VSV / ASV • SIMV • CPAP • Automode • ATC

Notes Page

4 Initial Settings

CONTENTS

Initial Settings Summary Chart 4-2

Initial Settings
Volumes 4-3
Rate 4-7
Inspiratory Pressures 4-8
PEEP 4-9
Oxygen 4-10
Times (T_I, T_E, I:E) 4-11
Flow (Rate, Waveform) 4-13
Sensitivity 4-14
Humidification 4-15
Alarms 4-16

Clinical Judgment Note:

This chapter has been created to give basic information on initial settings for Invasive Ventilation. Obviously it would be nearly impossible to account for every clinical condition, disease process, comorbidities, etc. This information, therefore, should be considered in context with the "whole picture" including systematic patient assessment.

Summary of Initial Settings

Initial settings should be based upon:

1. **Foundation Settings**: Generic Settings that take into account safety and basic physiology (such as anatomic deadspace).
2. **Patient-Specific Titration**: A combination of evidence-based support and clinical experience which takes into account patho-physiology, mechanics, patient age and size, and ventilator aspects. See Disease Chapter for specific recommendations.

Initial Settings Overview

Parameter	Suggested Range	Brief Notes
Minute Ventilation $\dot{V}_E$	5-10 L/min	Occasionally set, but should always be clinically monitored
V_T	6-8 cc/kg IBW	8 cc/kg IBW is common starting point
f	12-20 (15) breaths/minute	15 breaths/min is common starting point
PIP	15 cmH_2O	Titrate to desired V_T range
PEEP	5 cmH_2O	Considered physiologic by most clinicians
T_I	0.8 - 1.2 sec	Set to maintain I:E ratio of about 1:2 - 1:3 (more directly depends on *f*)
$\dot{V}_I$	40 - 100 L/min	
waveform	Constant (De-celerating when possible)	Not all modes allow you to set the flow waveform
FIO_2	0.50 or 1.0	Two strategies - either start moderate and titrate, or start at 1.0 and wean
Trigger	Flow (preferred) 1-3 L/min	

VOLUMES

Minute Ventilation ($\dot{V}_E$)*	
Initial Setting	5 - 10 L/min (in modes where minute ventilation is a set variable)

*Sometimes abbreviated MV

Calculations

Patient making no effort in A/C or other control modes:

$f \times V_T$

With Spontaneous Modes:

Minute Ventilation is calculated by averaging return tidal volumes by total rate.

SIMV $\dot{V}_E$ = [SET f x Set V_T (or return V_T)] + [Spont f x Spont V_T]

Notes:

$\dot{V}_E$ is the major determinant of Alveolar Ventilation ($\dot{V}_A$) which determines $PaCO_2$

($\dot{V}_E \approx 1/PaCO_2$):

↑ $\dot{V}_E$ to ↓ $PaCO_2$

↓ $\dot{V}_E$ to ↑ $PaCO_2$

Determining factors for selecting appropriate $\dot{V}_E$ include target pH, $PaCO_2$, spontaneous ventilation, and disease state

Calculation of Normal $\dot{V}_E$

Males: $\dot{V}_E$ = 4 x BSA

Females: $\dot{V}_E$ = 3.5 x BSA

Initial Settings

Tidal Volume (V_T)	
Initial Setting	5-8 cc/kg IBW

- Regardless of Actual Body Weight (ABW), tidal volumes should be set based on Ideal Body Weight (IBW)
- Clinically, V_T is usually "set and forget", though it may be altered (usually ↓) occasionally in response to Pplat, auto-PEEP, VI, disease state, tubing compliance, spontaneous ventilation, and synchrony/comfort
- VT may go as low as 4 cc/kg, and occasionally as high as 10 cc/kg.

See chart on back of front cover for quick reference numbers

Quick Formula (Calculating IBW for V_T from lbs)

Female IBW (lbs) = 100 + 5 [Ht (in) - 60]
Male IBW (lbs) = 106 + 6 [Ht (in) - 60]

IBW (kg) = IBW (lbs) / 2.2

Quick Formula (Calculating IBW for V_T from kgs)

Female IBW (kgs) = 45.5 kg + 2.3(Ht [in] - 60)
Male IBW (kgs) = 50 kg + 2.3(Ht [in] - 60)

Note: Estimating Height of Patients in a bed is often inaccurate. Patients should be measured with a measuring tape.

Factors Affecting Delivered V_T during Volume Ventilation

1) Tubing Compliance

V_T (delivered to patient) = V_T (set) – CCV (circuit compressible volume)

CCV = volume loss to tubing compliance

= CF (compliance factor of tubing) x $P_{gradient}$

= CF (mL/cm H_2O) x (PIP – PEEP)

Determining CF

Set ventilator V_T to 100-200 cc, set pressure limit as high as possible, completely occlude patient wye connection, manually cycle ventilator, record expired V_T (mL) and PIP (cm H_2O);

CF = V_T /PIP.

Clinical Notes

CCV may then be added to V_T (set) to achieve V_T (desired), if different from V_T (delivered). (Newer ventilators automatically compensate for this tubing loss). Correcting for tubing compliance loss is especially important in infants, children and very small patients when V_T is < 300 mL.

2) Mechanical Deadspace

VD_{mech} (mechanical deadspace) is usually insignificant: HME's add ≈ 20 - 90 cc. Wye connectors add ≈ 75 cc and ET tubes deduct ≈ 75 cc (1 cc/kg) so these two cancel each other out.

Determining V_T Delivery during Pressure Ventilation

How To Set Pressure

Option 1	Option 2
1) Volume ventilate with desired V_T to find P_{plat} and EEP. 2) Set PIP at Pplat and baseline pressure at EEP. 3) Adjust PIP as needed to obtain desired V_T.	1) Start at low PIP (10-15 cm H_2O) and check V_T. 2) Adjust PIP as needed to obtain desired V_T.

V_T ≈ PIP - PEEP (PEEP includes any auto-PEEP)

P_{plat} = P_{alv} ≈ peak Palv *It is recommended that a maximum Pplat of 30 cm H_2O is not exceeded.*

Initial Settings

Factors Affecting Delivered V_T during Pressure Ventilation

Pressure Gradient (PIP - PEEP)	Patient's Lungs	T_I
↑ PIP – PEEP → ↑ V_T ↓ PIP – PEEP → ↓ V_T ↑ auto-PEEP → ↓ V_T	↓ CL → ↓ V_T ↑ CL → ↑ V_T ↓ Raw → ↑ V_T ↑ Raw → ↓ V_T	↑ T_I → ↑ V_T (with active flow) ↓ T_I → ↓ V_T

Concerns with Improperly Set V_T

Concern	V_T Limit	Consequence
V_T too HIGH	≥ 8-10 (or more) cc/kg IBW	Volutrauma Barotrauma (indirectly)
V_T too LOW	≤ 4 (or less) cc/kg IBW	Anatomic Dead-space means alevolar ventilation is not effectively occurring

Ventilator Rate (f)	
Initial Setting	12 - 20 breaths/minute

Quick Formula (Calculating New f to alter $PaCO_2$)
New Rate (f) = $\frac{\text{Current Rate} \times \text{Current } PaCO_2}{\text{Desired } PaCO_2}$

$f = \dot{V}_E / V_T$
$f = 60 / T_I + T_E$

*Note that altering f also alters I:E ratio (or T_I and T_E if I:E ratio is set), so the clinician should take care to double-check those other parameters when altering f.

Rate is the primary control for altering pH and $PaCO_2$:
↑ f to ↑pH and ↓$PaCO_2$
↓ f to ↓pH and ↑ $PaCO_2$

CLINICAL NOTES:

- Permissive hypercapnia may be needed in some disease states (e.g., ARDS) to keep Pplat < 30 - 35 cm H_2O.
- Determining factors for selecting appropriate rate include: target $PaCO_2$, pH, V_T, PIP, $\dot{V}_I$, PEEP, auto-PEEP, mode, C_L, Raw, V_D/V_T, metabolic rate, spontaneous ventilation, and patient comfort.
- For disorders requiring lower V_T (such as ARDS), higher f may be required to maintain an adequate $\dot{V}_E$.
- For obstructive disorders, a lower f may be required to allow for sufficient expiratory time (to avoid or relieve air trapping), sometimes as much as allowing for an overall I:E ratio of 1:6.

Note: Usually f refers to frequency, and is the set rate of the ventilator. RR refers to the patient's rate and is not used consistently: sometimes it is used to mean spontaneous patient rate, and other times it is used to mean total ventilator + spontaneous rate.

Initial Settings

Inspiratory Pressure (IP, PIP, P_{peak})	
Initial Setting	~ 15 cmH_2O (above PEEP*) (titrate PIP to deliver 6-8 cc/kg IBW)

* Two types of ventilator settings:

1. PIP = the pressure above PEEP (PIP - PEEP)
2. PIP = total pressure (PIP + PEEP)

CLINICAL NOTES:

Inspiratory Pressure should be set in context to the patient's underlying state. The goal is usually to maintain $P_{Plat} < 30\ cmH_2O$.

Permissive hypercapnia may be needed in some disease states in order to accomplish this goal.

Positive End Expiratory Pressure (PEEP)	
Initial Setting	~ 5 cmH_2O is considered **physiologic** > 5 cmH_2O is viewed as **therapeutic**

Most clinicians recommend physiologic PEEP as a baseline to maintain Functional Residual Capacity (FRC) (exception: APRV).

For Therapeutic application:

Indications:

$PaO_2 \leq 60$ mmHg -or-
$SaO_2 \leq 90$ % on $F_IO_2 \geq 0.5$

Contraindications:

Excessive PIP, Pplat > 30 cm H_2O, hypotension, untreated pneumothorax, ↑ICP, large bronchopleural fistula, and possibly unilateral lung disease or COPD

Determining factors for selecting PEEP include: F_IO_2, target PaO_2, CL, and hemodynamic response.

Subsequent changes are based on ABGs, F_IO_2 needs, PEEP tolerance, auto-PEEP, trigger asynchrony, and hemodynamic response.

See PEEP Topics in Management Chapter for further discussion, including Optimal PEEP.

Fraction of Inspired Oxygen (F_IO_2)	
Initial Setting*	0.50, then titrate per SpO_2 / PaO_2 OR 1.0, then wean quickly, as clinically able

*If Baseline ABG is available, and PaO_2 is in desired range, use similar F_IO_2. If PaO_2 is not in desired range, use the following formula:

Quick Formula (Calculating New F_IO_2 to alter PaO_2)
New F_IO_2 $= \dfrac{\text{Desired } PaO_2 \times \text{Current } F_IO_2}{\text{Current } PaO_2}$

- Initial F_IO_2 must be evaluated by ABG (PaO_2) after patient stabilization, and adjusted.
- Any further adjustment needed is most likely due to MV effects on cardiopulmonary function.
- ↓ to < 0.5 as soon as clinically indicated. If F_IO_2 > 0.65 is required, consider PEEP.
- Determining factors for selecting appropriate F_IO_2 include target PaO_2, PEEP, $\overline{P}aw$, and hemodynamic status.

P_AO_2 Targets

Normal lung	≥ 80 mmHg
Mild lung injury	≥ 70 mmHg
Moderate lung injury	≥ 60 mmHg
Severe lung injury	≥ 55 mmHg

Inspiratory Time (T_I)	
Initial Setting	0.8 - 1.2 sec *

* Note that the actual T_I is less important than the resulting I:E ratio, so be sure to calculate and assess I:E ratio after making a change.

In Volume Modes, T_I is the result of $V_T/\dot{V}_I$ so even when set as a parameter, changing T_I will alter the flowrate ($\downarrow T_I = \uparrow \dot{V}_I$)

In Pressure Modes, T_I is a directly set parameter. Changing TI will alter the amount of time available for volume to build ($\uparrow T_I = \uparrow V_T$)

Determining factors for selecting appropriate T_I include oxygenation, rate, auto-PEEP, hemodynamic status, CL, Raw, patient-ventilator synchrony, and lung recruitment.

Expiratory Time (T_E)	
Initial Setting	Indirectly Set (T_I and *f*)

Usually a function of T_I and *f*.

$T_E = (60 / f) - T_I$

Remember, Expiratory Time is PASSIVE in most modes of ventilation (meaning TI receives priority, and whatever is left for the breath's cycle is for expiration). The exception to this is with High Frequency Oscillatory Ventilation (HFOV) where expiratory time is active.

Inspiratory:Expiratory Ratio (I:E Ratio)	
Initial Setting	1:2 - 1:3*

*I:E ratio may be a directly set parameter, or may be the function of other set parameters (f and T_I often)

Determining factors for selecting appropriate I:E ratio include hemodynamic response to MV, oxygenation status, patient-ventilator synchrony.

Small I:E ratios (longer T_E: 1:4, 1:6) may be used for patients requiring longer exhalation to avoid air-trapping and auto-PEEP (e.g., asthma, COPD).

Large I:E ratios (longer T_I: 1:1, 1:2) may be used for patients requiring ↑ $\overline{P}aw$ and ↑ gas distribution time.

Inverse I:E ratios should not be used until traditional MV strategies have failed to improve patient's ventilation and oxygenation.

$\dot{V}_I$:	↑ $\dot{V}_I$ → ↓T_I →smaller I:E ratio ↓ $\dot{V}_I$ → ↑T_I → larger I:E ratio
V_T:	↑ V_T → ↑ T_I → larger I:E ratio ↓ V_T → ↓ T_I → smaller I:E ratio
f:	↑ RR → ↓ T_E → larger I:E ratio ↓ RR → ↑ T_E → smaller I:E ratio
T_I %:	↑ TI% → larger I:E ratio (see →

T_I%	I:E Ratio
14.3%	1:6
16.7%	1:5
20.0%	1:4
25.0%	1:3
33.3%	1:2
50.0%	1:1
60.0%	1.5:1
66.7%	2:1

Inspiratory Flow Rate ($\dot{V}_I$)	
Initial Setting	40 - 100 L/min (Volume Modes)

Goal:

- Set $\dot{V}_I \geq$ patient's peak inspiratory demand and deliver a target I:E ratio (See I:E Ratio for more information)
- Assess Pressure Scalar or P-V Loop (see Waveform Graphics Chapter) to ensure goal is met

Minimum $\dot{V}_I = \dot{V}_E \times (I + E)$

ARDS: slow $\dot{V}_I$ (T_I of 3-4 time constants)
COPD: fast $\dot{V}_I$ (T_E of 3-4 time constants) (avoid too high a flow)

Slower flow rates may decrease PIP and improve gas distribution, but also increase the risk of air-trapping, cardiovascular side effects, and may lead to flow starvation. Faster flow rates may meet patient demand, decreasing WOB and air-trapping, but may result in an increased PIP and less effective gas distribution.

Inspiratory Flow Waveform	
Initial Setting	There is some debate in initial flow pattern, but Decelerating Flow is generally recommended in Volume modes. Pressure modes, by default, utilize decelerating flow

$\dot{V}$ with a decelerating waveform may provide similar results to PV. PV has a true decelerating flow, but in VV, the decelerating flow is algorithm-driven, which can lead to "flow starvation".
Changing flow patterns may affect peak $\dot{V}_I$, T_I and/or T_E, depending on the ventilation type.

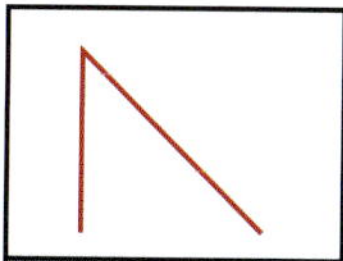
Decelerating Flow

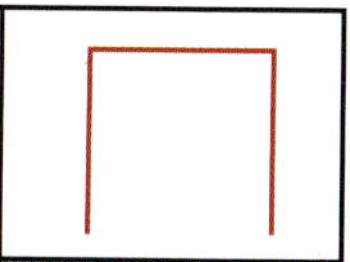
Square Flow

There are additional patterns (Sinusoidal, Accelerating), but they are not typically used clinically, so are not included here.

Sensitivity (Inspiratory Trigger)	
Initial Setting	Flow (preferred): 1-3 L/min or as sensitive as possible without causing auto-triggering Pressure: 0.5 - 2.0 cmH_2O below baseline

- Fine-tune the setting to prevent auto-triggering, ↑ WOB, and/or patient-ventilator asynchrony
- Observe patient's inspiratory efforts, pressure manometer, and graphics display

If auto-PEEP (PEEPI) is present:

- Pressure triggering = $PEEP_I$ + (- 0.5 to - 2.0 cm H_2O)
- Adjust $PEEP_E$ (set PEEP) to equal and cancel out $PEEP_I$

Example: If auto-PEEP is 10 cm H_2O, the pt. must generate - 11 to - 12 cm H_2O to trigger ventilator. ↑ $PEEP_E$ until pt. effectively triggers the ventilator (up to 80% of auto-PEEP) (e.g., 8 cm H_2O).

See Ventilator Graphics: trigger asynchrony and auto-PEEP.

Measuring auto-PEEP (PEEPI):

1) *Measure*: See Ch 11.
2) *Estimate*:
   a) ↑ $PEEP_E$ until PIP begins to rise
   b) ↑ $PEEP_E$ until accessory muscle use decreases
   c) ↑ $PEEP_E$ until each inspiratory effort triggers the ventilator

Note: If sensitivity is too sensitive, the ventilator will auto-cycle. If sensitivity is too insensitive, there will be an ↑ WOB.

Initial Settings

Sensitivity (Inspiratory Cycle Off, Expiratory Sensitivity)	
Initial Setting	25% For PS Breaths. This means that the breath will cycle off at 25% of Peak Inspiratory Flow

Adjust down to 10% for Restrictive; up to 40% for obstructive disorder

Humidification	
Initial Setting	Varies by hospital, most evidence is inconclusive on which type: HME (passive or active) - OR - Active Humidifier 37° Celsius

Invasive Ventilation

Replace HME at least every 1-5 days, or per manufacturer, and as indicated (soiled, etc.)

If using a passive HME, consider switching to heated humidity when*:

- Patients have thick and/or copious secretions
- Loss of V_T (leak in patient or cuff)
- Low V_T strategies (ARDS)
- In difficult-to-wean patients
- Hypothermic patients (Temp < 32° C)
- High Minute Ventilations (> 10 L/min)

***Summarized from AARC Clinical Practice Guidelines, 2012**

Noninvasive Ventilation:

- Use of HME is generally not recommended
- See Noninvasive Chapter for more details

Ventilator Alarms		
Initial Settings	**Alarm**	**Setting**
	Apnea	< 20 sec
	High/Low $\dot{V}_E$	10-15% +/- set $\dot{V}_E$
	High/Low V_T	10-15% +/- set V_T
	High/Low PIP	10 cmH_20 +/- avg. PIP
	High/Low PEEP	3-5 cmH_20 +/- set PEEP
	High/Low F_IO_2	5% +/- set F_IO_2
	High/Low Rate	10-15 bpm +/- set rate
	I:E Ratio	when I>E
	Temp	2° above/below set temp.

Typical Problems:

Problem	Consequence
Alarms set too sensitive	Results in alarms that activate too often, resulting in alarm fatigue. Alarm fatigue occurs when hospital staff become desensitized to alarms and may become less likely to respond to a legitimate alarm event
Alarms set too wide (not sensitive enough)	Results in the clinician being unaware of key changes in the patient's condition

Notes Page

Notes Page

5 Assessment and Troubleshooting

CONTENTS

Sudden Patient Distress Algorithm 5-3
Patient Problems 5-4
Ventilator Problems 5-5

Selected Assessments
Arterial Blood Gases 5-6
Oxygenation (Internal, External) 5-7
Ventilation 5-8
Ventilatory Mechanics 5-9
  Load 5-9
  Capacity 5-9
  Static Compliance 5-10
  Dynamic Compliance 5-10
  Airway Resistance 5-11

Ventilator Assessment
Checklist 5-12
Troubleshooting 5-13
Changes in Tidal Volume 5-13
Changes in Minute Ventilation 5-13
Changes in Respiratory Rate 5-14
Changes in Pressures (PIP, PEEP, etc.) 5-14
  Checking for Leaks 5-15
Changes in I:E Ratio 5-16
Loss of Power 5-16
Gas Supply Issues 5-16
Patient-Ventilator Asynchrony 5-17

Make It Your Own

Notes Page

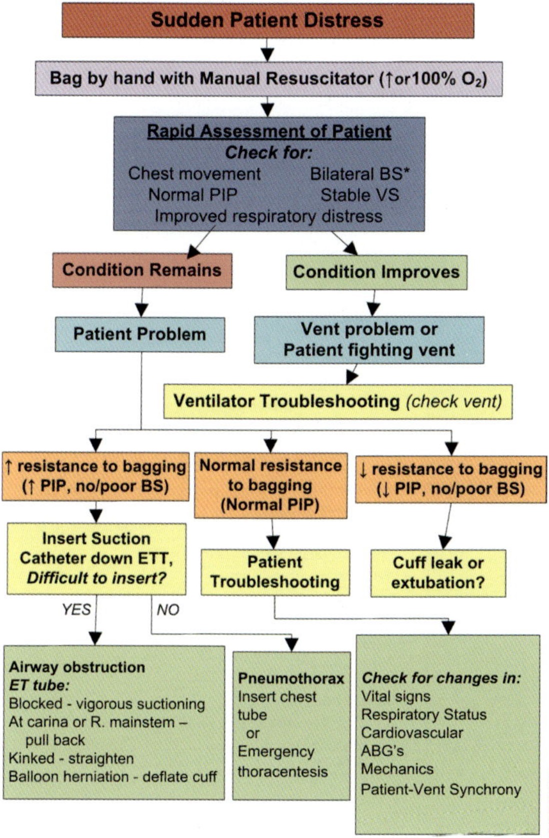

* Check for presence of breath sounds, adventitious breath sounds, and intensity of breath sounds during this rapid assessment.

Patient Problems	
Assess for:	
Airway Patency	• Attempt to pass suction catheter • Consider instilling Normal Saline • Check for kinks/biting of ET tube

ET Tube	• Verify ET Tube placement:
	  • Right Mainstem
	  • Partial Extubation
	• Cuff Herniation, Leak, Rupture

Tension PTX	• Consider if difficult to ventilate patient (by bagging patient, or sudden ↑ in PIP)

Synchrony	• Verify sedation status
	  • Pain
	  • Stress
	• Watch for pt effort against ventilator behavior

Broncho-spasm	• Auscultate
Cardiovas-cular	• Fluid (auscultate) • Innominate Artery Rupture (Over-inflate Cuff if sudden, large amt of frank blood) • Pulmonary Embolism
Change in V/Q	• Change in patient position recently? • Atelectasis • Air Trapping
Other Causes	• Abdominal Distension • Drug or Alcohol withdrawal

Ventilator Problems	
If any doubt about the ventilator, the patient must be taken off the ventilator and manually ventilated in order to isolate patient problems from ventilator issues.	
Synchrony	Verify mode and parameters are appropriate for patient: • Trigger/Sensitivity (too sensitive, not sensitive enough) • Inappropriate Support (too much, too little) • Inadequate F_IO_2 (hypoxemia)
Ventilator Leaks	• Check for leak/disconnect (patient and ventilator side)
Ventilator Obstructions	• Check ventilator filters and tubing for water • Check HME patency (secretions, water) • Verify exhalation valve is working (particularly when administering nebulized drugs) • If inline suction, verify suction catheter is in appropriate position in sheath (not obstructing ET Tube)

If any doubt about ventilator function exists, attempt to briefly troubleshoot. If the problem persists, strong consideration should be given to swapping out for a new ventilator.

Arterial Blood Gases

Value (art, mix ven), unit	Arterial		Mixed Venous	
	Norm	Range	Norm	Range
pH (pHa, pH$\bar{v}$), units	7.40	7.35-7.45	7.36	7.31-7.41
PCO_2 ($PaCO_2$, $P\bar{v}CO_2$), mmHg	40	35-45	46	41-51
PO_2 (PaO_2, $P\bar{v}O_2$), mmHg	100	80-100	40	35-42
O_2 Sat (SaO_2, $S\bar{v}O_2$), %	97%	95-100%	75%	68-77%
HCO_3, mEq/L	24	22-26	24	22-26
TCO_2	25	23-27	25	23-27
BE, mEq/L	0	+/- 2	0	+/- 2
O_2 content (CaO_2, $C\bar{v}O_2$), mL/dL	20	15-24	15	12-15

See Oakes' ***ABG Pocket Guide*** for in-depth coverage of ABG Interpretation, including differential diagnosis of ABG disorders.

Oxygenation at the Lungs (external respiration)			Oxygenation at the Tissues (internal respiration)		
Measure	**Norm**	**Ab-norm**	**Measure**	**Norm**	**Ab-norm**
Adequacy					
PaO_2*	80-100 mmHg	< 80 mmHg	**$P\bar{V}O_2$**	35-42 mmg	< 35 or > 45 mmHg
CaO_2	15-24 mL/dL	↑↓	**$C\bar{V}O_2$**	12-15 mL/dL	↑↓
SaO_2**	> 95%	< 95%	**$S\bar{V}O_2$**	60-80%	< 60%
SpO_2	> 95%	< 95%	**$Ca\text{-}\bar{V}O_2$**	4.5-5.0 mL/dL	↑↓
Efficiency					
$PA\text{-}aO_2$	10-25 mmHg (air) 30-50 mmHg (100%)	>25 mmHg	**$O_{2_{ER}}$**	25%	↑↓
			$\dot{V}O_2$	200 - 250 mL/min	↑↓
			$\dot{D}O_2$	750 - 1000 mL/min	↑↓
PaO_2/PAO_2	0.8-0.9	<0.6	**VQI**	0.8	↑↓
PaO_2/FIO_2	>300	<300			
$PA\text{-}aO_2/PaO_2$	<1.0	>1.0			
Q_S/Q_T phys	2-5%	> 20%			

*Normal Variations: Due to age, FIO_2, or barometric pressure
Age: $PaO_2 \approx 110$ - 1/2 patient's age

**SaO_2 = calculated O_2 saturation from PaO_2
SpO_2 = Peripheral O_2 saturation - measured value of Hgb

Assessment of Ventilation

	Normal	Abnormal		Normal	Abnormal
Adequacy			**Efficiency**		
$\dot{V}_E$	5-10 L/min	↑↓	**V_D phys**	1/3$\dot{V}$E	↑↓
$PaCO_2$	35-45 mmHg	↑↓	**V_D/V_T**	0.33-0.45	↑↓
$P_{ET}CO_2$	35-43 mmHg (4.6 - 5.6%)	↑↓			
$Pa\text{-}_{ET}CO_2$	1-5 mmHg	> 6 mmHg			

Changes in Ventilation

Hyperventilation - Causes of	Hypoventilation - Causes of
• Anxiety • CNS pathology • Hypoxia • Metabolic acidosis (DKA, etc.) • Mech. Ventilation (settings) • Pain • Physical Therapy (Exercise)	• Mechanical Ventilation • Neuropathy • N-M blockade (disease, blocking agents) • Respiratory center depression (pathologic, iatrogenic) • Respiratory muscle weakness (fatigue,disease) • Trauma

Assessment of Ventilatory Mechanics

Assessment of Load

	Normal	Abnormal
Adequacy:		
C_{dyn}	40-60 mL/cmH_2O	↓
C_{stat}	70-100 mL/cmH_20	↓
Raw	0.5 - 2.5 cmH_20/L/sec @ 0.5 L/sec (4-8 with ET tube)	> 15 cmH_2O/L/sec
RSBI (f/V_T)	< 105*	> 105

*See RSBI in Weaning Chapter for more information on typical values

Assessment of Capacity

	Normal	Abnormal
Respiratory Drive:		
P0.1	< 2 cm H_2O	> 4-6 cmH_2O
Respiratory Muscle Strength		
VC	60-80 mL/kg	< 60 mL/kg
P_Imax (MIP, NIF)	< -60 cmH_2O	> -30 cmH_20
Respiratory Muscle Endurance		
MVV	120-180 L/min	< 20 L/min
$\dot{V}_E$/MVV	< 1:2	> 1:2

Changes in Ventilatory Mechanics

Static Compliance

<table>
<tr><th colspan="2">Conditions Causing ↓ Cstat</th><th>Conditions Causing ↑ Cstat</th></tr>
<tr><td><u>Lung</u>
• Air-trapping (auto-PEEP)
• ARDS
• Atelectasis
• Bronchial intubation
• Consolidation
• Fibrosis
• Hemothorax,
• Pleural effusion,
• Pneumonia
• Pneumothorax
• Position change
• Pulmonary edema</td><td><u>Thorax/diaphragm</u>
• Abdominal distension
• Ankylosing spondylitis
• Kyphoscoliosis
• Muscle tension
• Obesity</td><td>• Improvement in disease state
• COPD (esp. emphysema)
• Flail chest
• Position change</td></tr>
</table>

Dynamic Compliance

Conditions Causing ↓ Cdyn	Conditions Causing ↑ Cdyn
• ↓Cstat (see above) • ↑ Raw (see below)	• ↑ Cstat (see above) • ↓ Raw (see below)

Airway Resistance Changes

Conditions Causing ↑ Raw

Obstruction of Airway	**Collapse of Airway**

• Condensation in circuit
• Epiglottitis
• ET tube
    • small diameter
    • plugging
    • kinking
    • biting
• Foreign body aspiration
• Mucosal edema
• Post intubation swelling
• Secretions
• Tumors
	• Asthma
	• Bronchospasm
	• Bronchitis
	• Bronchiolitis
	• Emphysema
	• Low lung volumes
	• Laryngotracheobronchitis (croup)
	• Pneumothorax
	• Pleural effusion
	• Tumors

High $\dot{V}_I$ (turbulence)	

Methods to Assist in ↓ Raw
• Bronchodilator therapy • Steroid administration (slower) • Improvement of an ↑ Raw • Suctioning • ↓ $\dot{V}_I$

Assess/Troubleshoot

Ventilator Assessment

Ventilator Settings		Ventilator Circuit
Orders: • Settings consistent with orders? • Verification of changes • Current Settings • Mode and breath type **Oxygenation**: • F_IO_2 (set, analyzed) **Volumes**: • V_T (set, delivered, expired) • V_T (spont) • $\dot{V}_E$ mach (set, delivered) • $\dot{V}_E$ spont • $\dot{V}_E$ total **Rate**: • *f* (set, delivered) • *f* (spont) **Pressures**: • PIP (Ppeak) • Pplat (Palv) • PTA (PIP – Pplat) • $\bar{P}aw$ • PEEP (set, auto) • CPAP • PS level • Pressure limits	**Sensitivity**: • Threshold (P or $\dot{V}$) • Patient triggering • Auto-triggering **Times**: • T_I • T_E • I/E **Flows**: • $\dot{V}_I$ • $\dot{V}_I$ waveform • $\dot{V}_I$ continuous **Sighs (if used):** • Volume • Rate • Frequency **Alarms** (set & functioning): • $\dot{V}_E$ (High/Low) • V_T (High/Low) • Pressure (High/Low) • F_IO_2 • PEEP (High/Low) • Rate (High/Low) **Graphics** See Vent Graphics Chapter for Assessment of graphics	**Humidifier**: • Temperature (set, measured) • Water level • HME (condition, changing) **Tubing**: • Circuit temp. • Condensate • Clean, secure • ET tube (tension, position, depth) • Tubing compliance • Circuit change (?) ***Circuit Changes should be changed when visibly soiled, or per manufacturer's guidelines. Frequent changing increases infection risk*** **Other** *Location/condition:* • Manual resuscitator with mask, tubing, and flowmeter, PEEP valve • Suction equipment (Pressure) • Chest tube apparatus

Ventilator Troubleshooting

Changes in Ventilator Parameters

Changes in Tidal Volume

↓ Inspired Tidal Volume	↑ Inspired Tidal Volume
Volume Ventilation: • If corresponding ↓ in PIP: see PIP (↓) • If not a corresponding ↓ in PIP = altered settings *Pressure Ventilation*: Above, plus ↓ C or ↑ Raw	*Volume Ventilation*: • If corresponding ↑ in PIP: see PIP (↑) • If not a corresponding ↑ in PIP =altered settings *Pressure Ventilation:* Above, plus ↑C or ↓ Raw

↓ Expired Tidal Volume	↑ Expired Tidal Volume

Volume Ventilation:
• If corresponding ↓ in PIP: See PIP ↓
• If not a corresponding ↓ in PIP:
  • Leak in spirometer, between exhalation valve and spirometer/transducer, or from chest tube
  • Malfunction of transducer
 	
Pressure Ventilation:
Above, plus ↓ C, ↑ Raw, or ↑ auto-PEEP
	Volume Ventilation:
	• If corresponding ↑ in PIP: see PIP ↑
	• If not a corresponding ↑ in PIP:
	  • Transducer malfunction
	  • External nebulizer flow
	
	Pressure Ventilation:
	Above, plus ↑C, ↓ Raw, or ↓ auto-PEEP

Changes in Minute Volume

↓or ↑ Minute Volume
Same as ↓ or↑ V_T (above) with the added effect of rate changes.

Changes in Rate (↑/↓ or Apnea)

Machine	Patient
• Altered settings • Inappropriate sensitivity • Malfunction/disconnection • Nebulizers (rate, trigger)	• See changes in Vital Signs (above) • Be particularly aware of pain/anxiety issues • Patient disconnection from ventilator (↓ or apnea)

Changes in Pressures

Slow Rise of Needle on Pressure Gauge to PIP	Slow Return of Needle on Pressure Gauge to Baseline
• Leak	• Exhalation tubing or exhalation valve tubing kinked • Sticky exhalation valve • Expiratory resistance or inflation hold "ON"

↓ PEEP/CPAP		↑ PEEP/CPAP	
Machine	*Patient*	*Machine*	*Patient*
• Altered settings • ↓ expiratory flow • Proximal Paw line occluded	• ↑ pt inspiratory flowrate	• Altered settings • ↑ expiratory flow	• Auto-PEEP • Patient-ventilator asynchrony

Assess/Troubleshoot

↓ PIP	↑ PIP
Machine: • Altered settings • Internal leak/power or gas source failure **Circuit**: • Disconnection • Leak (see below) • Proximal Paw line occluded **Patient**: *CL* ↑: improved lung, position change *Raw* ↓: ↓ secretions or bronchospasm Patient-ventilator asynchrony (see below) *Leak at:* • ET tube (displaced in pharynx or esophagus) • Cuff (deflation/rupture/leak or inadequate inflation) • Chest tube • T-E fistula	**Machine**: • Altered settings • Blocked exhalation • Internal problem • Malfunctioning I or E valves **Circuit**: • Tubing kinked • H_2O in circuit **Patient**: • Auto-PEEP • *CL* ↓: abdominal distension, ARDS, atelectasis, hemothorax, pleural effusion, pneumonia, pneumothorax, position change, pulmonary edema • *Raw* ↑: bronchospasm, cough, edema, ET tube displaced (in RT mainstem, against carina), kinked, or bitten, ET tube cuff herniation, H_2O in circuit, secretions or mucous plugs. • Patient-ventilator asynchrony

Checking for Leaks

1. ***Check Patient***

   Remove patient from ventilator and manually ventilate.
   Listen to breath sounds over trachea.
   ET tube cuff inflated?

2. ***Check Ventilator:***

   Obstruct patient wye and manually cycle the ventilator.
   If the high pressure alarm fails to activate (in volume modes), obstruct the patient circuit at various places starting at the ventilator and working distal to find the leak (until the alarm does not activate).

I:E Ratio (↑ or ↓)

Machine	Patient
• Altered settings • Too sensitive or subtle leak	• Pressure cycling off (↑Raw) • Fighting the vent

Loss of Power or Low Gas Source - Check:

Electrical power supply:	*Gas supply:*
• Power switch on • Connection to outlet/battery • Fuse/circuit breaker • Reset button • **If any doubt about ventilator electrical function, take out of service**	• 50 psi wall connection or air compressor • Zone Valve • High pressure hose connections (patency of high pressure hoses; not crushed by bed wheels)

All life-saving equipment should be plugged into outlets connected to back-up systems (generators) - typically these outlets are red.

Specific plans should be in place in case of either red-outlet (generator) failure, or in those facilities without the outlets.

Portable cylinders should be readily available in case of failure of gas supply system.

Ventilator Inoperative: Take patient off ventilator, turn the ventilator off and reset. Be sure to run through pre-use check if available. **If any doubt at this point, take ventilator out of service.**

I:E Ratio Alarm

Usually I:E > 1:1 (correct settings)
If desired, check flowrate (VV)

F_IO_2 Error

Analyzer: uncalibrated or defective
Blender: source gas failure, tubing kinked, leak or disconnect

Patient-Ventilator Asynchrony ("Fighting the Vent")*

* See Ventilator Management, Chapter 8, for corrective actions

Potential Causes

Machine:

1) Triggering too sensitive
2) ↑ patient WOB:
   - Inadequate $\dot{V}_I$
   - Level of ventilator support inadequate
   - Prolonged T_I (VV) or flow cycle (PV)
   - Triggering too insensitive (setting or demand valve)
   - ↑ $\dot{V}_I$ resistance:
     - Bubble humidifier or water-laden HME
     - ET tube resistance (too small, kinks, secretions)
     - ↑ $\dot{V}_E$ (PEEP valve resistance)

Patient: Auto-PEEP, ↑ patient ventilatory drive, anxiety/stress

Make It Your Own

Notes Page

6 Ventilator Graphics

CONTENTS

Definition 6-3
Purposes (Indications) 6-3

Types of Graphics
Scalars
Pressure-Time 6-4
Volume-Time 6-7
Flow-Time 6-9
Loops
Pressure-Volume 6-11
Flow-Volume 6-14

Normal Graphics
Scalars
Pressure-Time 6-16
Volume-Time 6-18
Flow-Time 6-20
Loops
Pressure-Volume 6-22
Flow-Volume 6-24

Abnormal Graphics
by Waveform Type
Scalars
Pressure-Time 6-26
Volume-Time 6-28
Flow-Time 6-29
Loops
Pressure-Volume 6-30
Flow-Volume 6-33

(Continued on Next Page)

CONTENTS

by Problem

Patient

Air-Trapping (auto-PEEP) 6-35
Airway Resistance Changes 6-38
Compliance Changes 6-41
Excessive (active) Exhalation 6-43
Partial Obstruction 6-44

Ventilator

Over-distension 6-45
Leaks 6-46
Rate (Cycle) Asynchrony 6-48
Flow Asynchrony (Flow Starvation) 6-49
Trigger Asynchrony (settings) 6-50
Trigger Asynchrony (auto-PEEP) 6-51

Other Applications 6-52

Definition

Waveforms are graphic representations of data collected by the ventilator that reflect patient-ventilator interaction.

Purpose (Indications)

Patient

- Monitor patient's disease pathology (C + Raw)
- Calculate respiratory mechanics (C + Raw)
- Assess patient's response to therapy (e.g., bronchodilators)

Ventilator

- Monitor ventilator function
- Fine tune ventilator parameters and modes to:
  - o Improve patient comfort
  - o Decrease WOB
  - o Optimize ventilation

Patient-Ventilator Interaction

Interpret, evaluate, and troubleshoot patient's response to the ventilator

Clinical Note:

When analyzing graphic waveforms, it is important to first look at the parameters and the scaling of each parameter. It is imperative that the mode is identified. A graphic that appears to be abnormal could be normal depending on the mode and breath type.

Each graphic waveform is idealized. There are a myriad of variations seen in the clinical setting (far beyond the scope of this book).

The goal in understanding and interpreting graphics is not to memorize shapes, but rather to understand how they are created and how they are affected by variables.

See the Equation of Motion (Mechanics): Chapter 7

Types Of Graphic Waveforms

Scalars – Graphic displays of **pressure**, **volume**, and **flow** over time.

Loops – Graphic displays of two parameters (**Pressure and Volume** or **Flow and Volume**) on a horizontal (x) axis and a vertical (y) axis. Time is not depicted on loops.

Scalars

Pressure -Time Waveform

Spontaneous breath:

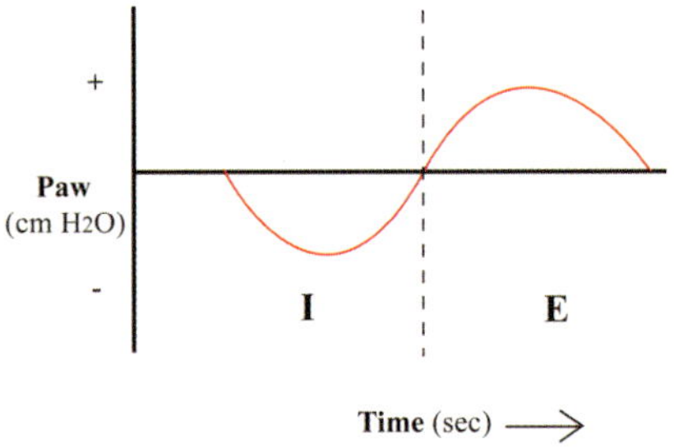

Ventilator breath:

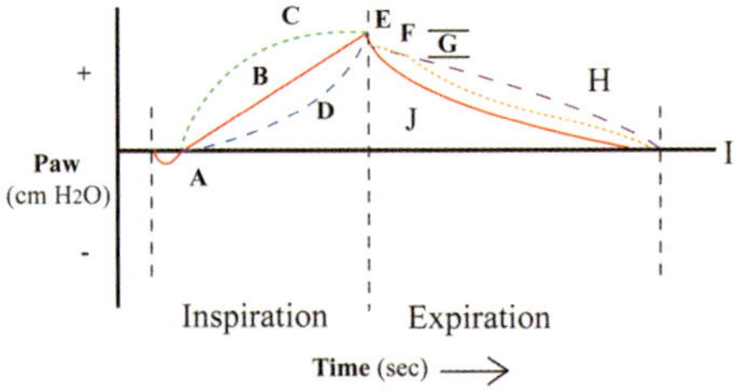

A No negative deflection = machine-triggered (MT) breath (controlled)

Negative deflection = patient-triggered (PT) breath (assisted)

The greater the depth and time below baseline, the greater the patient effort required to trigger the ventilator.

Flow-triggering (flow-by) will virtually eliminate patient effort, resulting in less negative deflection.

B Square wave inspiratory flow pattern

The steeper the slope, the greater the $\dot{V}_I$

C Decelerating inspiratory flow pattern

D Sine wave inspiratory flow pattern

E Peak inspiratory pressure (Ppeak)

Ppeak may rise to a plateau when a breath is pressure-controlled (limited) or pressure-supported. This Ppeak pressure plateau is not to be confused with Pplat.

Used to calculate Cdyn.

F Plateau pressure (Pplat)

Results from an inspiratory hold

Used to calculate Cstat

G Ppeak - Pplat = Raw (Raw is flow dependent)

Pressure required to overcome resistance of airway and ET tube.

H Expiratory retard

Analogous to pursed-lip breathing

May be patient-induced (e.g., COPD) or machine-induced (rarely done)

I Baseline pressure (beginning and end-expiratory pressure)

ZEEP – zero (atmospheric)

PEEP – positive (above zero)

NEEP – negative (below zero) (caution—indicates an abnormal pressure gradient)

Failure of the pressure curve to return to the set baseline pressure before the next inspiration = inadequate TE and may result in air-trapping and auto-PEEP

J Area under the entire curve, including any PEEP, is ≈ average $\overline{P}aw$.

Applications – Pressure-time waveforms are used to analyze:

Patient	Ventilator	Pt-Vent Interaction
• Air-trapping (auto-PEEP) • Airway obstruction • Active exhalation • Bronchodilator response • Respiratory mechanics (C + Raw)	• Breath type • Ppeak • Pplat • PEEP/CPAP • $\dot{V}_I$ • Pressure waveform shape • T_I, T_E, I:E	• Asynchrony • Triggering effort

Volume-Time Waveform

Spontaneous breath:

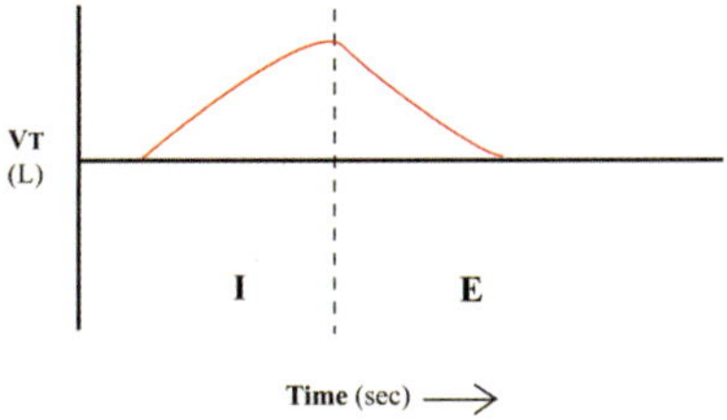

Ventilator breath:

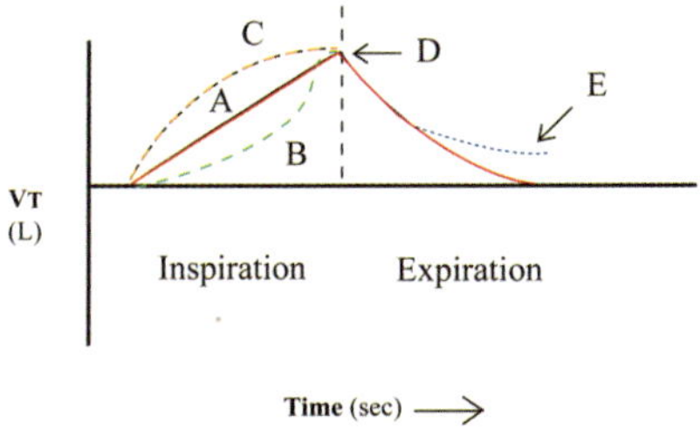

A	Square wave inspiratory flow pattern
B	Sine wave inspiratory flow pattern
C	Decelerating inspiratory flow pattern (or pressure-supported breath)
D	Inspiratory V_T (a plateau at this peak of the curve may indicate pressure-controlled or supported breath)
E	**An exhalation curve that does not return to baseline may indicate leak or air-trapping**

Waveform Graphics

Application – Volume-Time waveforms are used to analyze:

Patient	Ventilator	Pt-Vent Interaction
• Air-trapping (auto-PEEP) • Active exhalation	• Breath type • Volume waveform shape • V_T • $\dot{V}_I$ • Leaks	• Asynchrony

Flow-Time Waveform

Spontaneous breath:

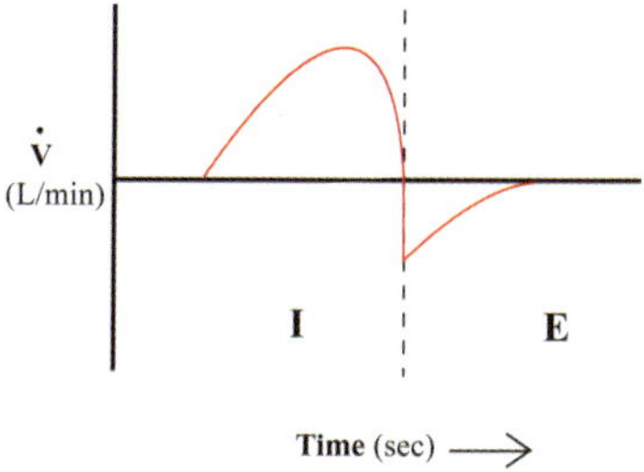

Ventilator breaths:

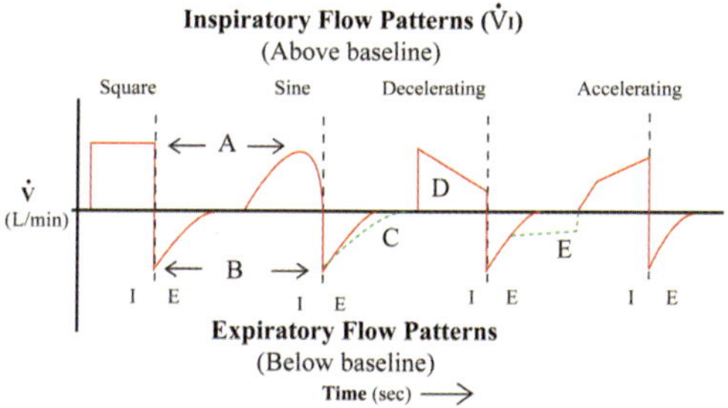

- **A** Peak inspiratory flow (set V̇I)
- **B** Peak expiratory flow
- **C** Expiratory retard—
  Increased resistance to expiratory flow (see H under pressure-time curve)
- **B/C** May be used to analyze response to bronchodilator therapy

continued next page

Waveform Graphics

D Pressure-control and supported breaths have a decelerating flow pattern

E Expiratory flow patterns have one basic shape and should return to baseline(zero flow) indicating a complete exhalation.

Expiratory flow that does not return to zero prior to the next inspiration, indicates inadequate T_E, resulting in air-trapping and auto-PEEP.

(The higher the end-expiratory flow, the greater the auto-PEEP)

An expiratory flow that returns to above the baseline indicates a leak during flow-by.

Applications – Flow-Time waveforms are used to analyze:

Patient	Ventilator	Pt-Vent Interaction
• Air-trapping (auto-PEEP) • Airway obstruction • Active exhalation • Bronchodilator response • Respiratory mechanics (C + Raw)	• Breath type • Flow waveform shape • Inspiratory flow • Flow starvation (VV) • Adjustment of inspiratory time in PV • Adjustment of rise to pressure time in PV • Leaks	• Asynchrony • Triggering effort

Volume-Pressure Loop

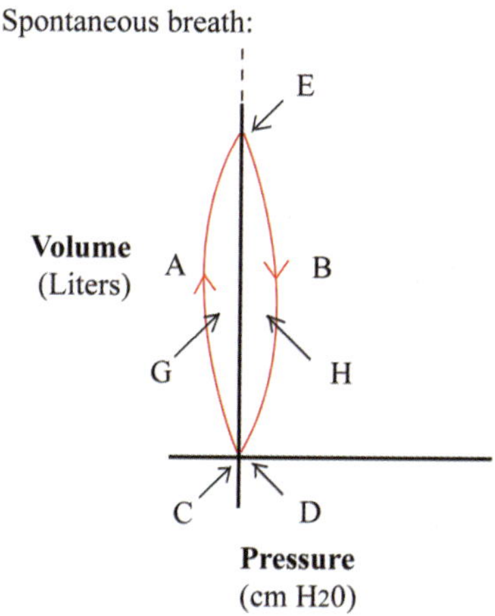

Ventilator Breath (Volume Ventilation)

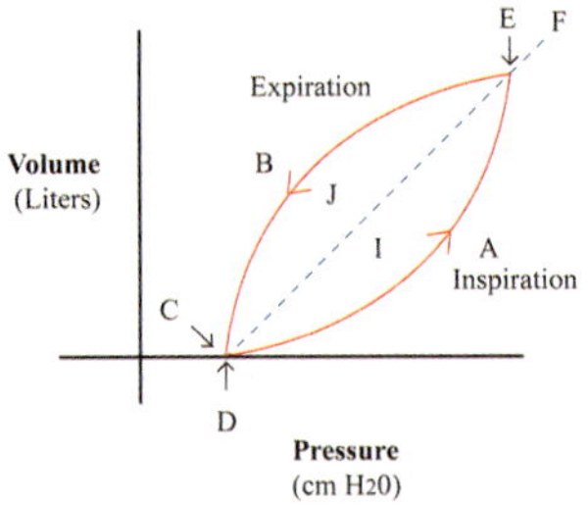

A Inspiratory curve (upward)

B Expiratory curve (downward)

Note: Spontaneous breaths go clockwise; positive pressure breaths always go counter clockwise.

C The bottom point of the loop:
Inspiration begins and expiration ends

D Point on pressure axis where inspiration (I) begins and expiration (E) ends (indicates end-expiratory pressure level)

E The upper point of the loop:
1) Inspiration ends and expiration begins
2) Point of maximal pressure and volume
3) Dynamic compliance ($\Delta V/\Delta P$)

F The imaginary (dashed) line between the 2 points (C & E), (begin I & end I) depicts the slope of the loop.
The slope is indicative of the patient's dynamic compliance ($\Delta V/\Delta P$)

G The area to the left of the vertical line represents patient inspiratory WOB (inspiratory resistance)

H The area to the right of the vertical axis represents patient expiratory WOB (expiratory resistance)

I The area of the curve to the right of the slope line depicts the ventilator WOB required to overcome Raw. (↑ area = ↑ work)
WOB = amount of pressure required to move a certain volume

J The area of the curve to the left of the slope line depicts the WOB required to overcome C_{RS}

Total WOB = area I and area J (↑ area = ↑ work)

Note: These areas show only the mechanical WOB by the ventilator and are only accurate if the patient is not contributing any WOB. Patient WOB can be measured indirectly by plotting the esophageal pressure.

Applications – Volume - Pressure loops are used to analyze:

Patient	Ventilator	Pt-Vent Interaction
• Airway obstruction • Active exhalation • Bronchodilator response • Lung over-distension • Respiratory mechanics • (Cdyn + Raw) • WOB	• Adjusting pressure support levels • Flow starvation (VV) • Leaks	• Triggering effort

Waveform Graphics

Flow-Volume Loop

Spontaneous breath:

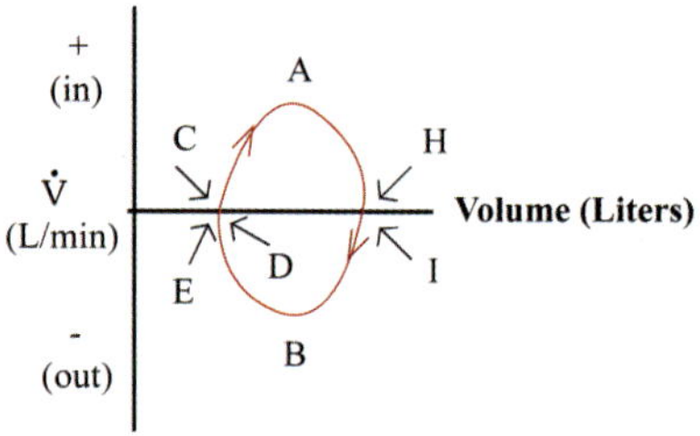

Ventilator breath:
(Volume Ventilation)

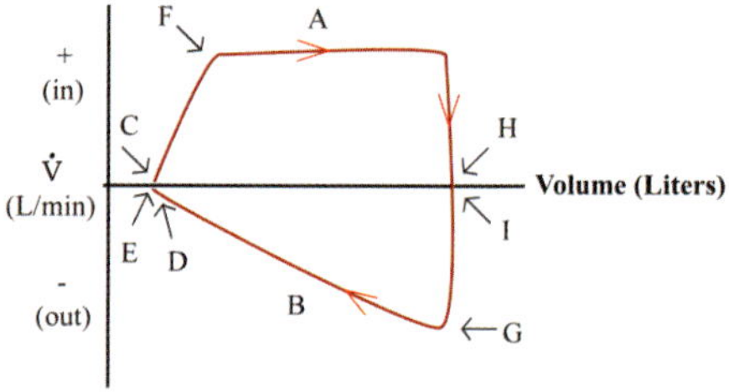

- **A** Inspiratory curve (above the horizontal axis)
  On the ventilator breath, the shape of the inspiratory curve will reflect the flow pattern set on the ventilator.
- **B** Expiratory curve (below the horizontal axis)
  The shape of the expiratory curve will reflect patient exhalation (usually passive).
- **C** Begin inspiration
- **D** End expiration
- **E** Point on volume axis where I begins and E ends. This indicates end-expiratory pressure level.
  Note: C, D, and E should all be the same point. (See abnormal waveforms if not)

F Peak inspiratory flow rate ($\dot{V}_I$)
G Peak expiratory flow rate
H Point on volume axis of maximum V_T and end I (flow rate 0)
I Begin E

Note: H and I should be the same point.
(See abnormal waveforms if not)

* **Note**:

Pulmonary function flow-volume loops (depicting FVC) traditionally display the inspiratory curve <u>below</u> the horizontal axis and expiration above the axis.

Ventilator flow-volume loops (depicting V_T) most commonly display the inspiratory curve <u>above</u> the horizontal axis and expiration below the axis (to maintain consistency with scalars).

There is, however, no set convention and some ventilators will display the loops like pulmonary function loops. When reading F-V loops, be certain to properly identify the orientation.

This book will display all loops with the inspiratory curve <u>above</u> the axis.

Applications – Flow-volume loops are used to analyze:

Patient	Ventilator	Pt-Vent Interaction
• Air-trapping (auto-PEEP) • Airway obstruction • Airway resistance changes • Active exhalation • Bronchodilator response	• Inspiratory flow • Expiratory flow • Flow starvation (VV) • V_T • Leaks • Water and secretions buildup	• Asynchrony

Normal Graphic Waveforms by Waveform Type

Scalars: Pressure-Time

Spontaneous Ventilation
During I, pressure is a negative deflection. During E, pressure is a positive deflection. Pressures are generally much lower than with ventilator breaths. I to E is patient-cycled

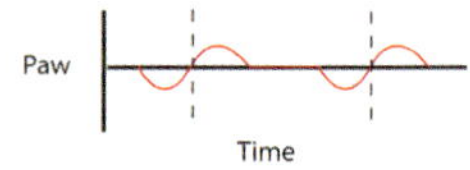

Volume Ventilation – Assist/Control (constant or square flow)
The pressure curve generally shows a linear rise to Ppeak. Ppeak is dependent on V_T, $\dot{V}_I$, PEEP, C, and Raw. 1st breath is assisted (patient-triggered). 2nd breath is controlled (machine-triggered). I to E is volume-cycled.

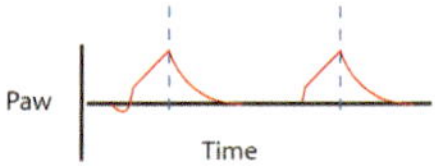

Clinical note: The pressure-time curve is the only scalar that identifies an assisted breath. The depth of deflection and the period of time below the baseline reflect the degree of patient effort to trigger the ventilator. Flow-triggering virtually eliminates all of the patient effort of triggering.

Volume Ventilation – Assist/Control (decelerating flow)
Same as square flow (above), except that the upward slope to Ppeak is usually convex.

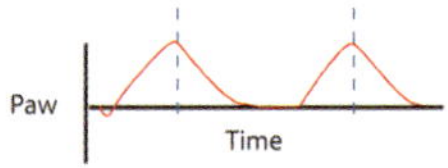

SIMV (square flow)
A combination of assisted VV and spontaneous ventilation.

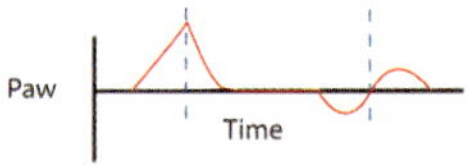

Pressure Ventilation – Assist/ Control	
The pressure curve generally shows an immediate rise to Ppeak (set pressure), which is then maintained during the entire inspiratory phase. The speed (slope) in which set pressure is reached is dependent on the ventilator (See rise to pressure time, Chapter 2, Operating Principles). Patient C and Raw generally do not affect the shape of the waveform. 1st breath is assisted (patient-triggered). 2nd breath is controlled (machine-triggered). I to E is time-cycled (hence T_I is constant). *Clinical note*: Ppeak = Pplat, provided there is zero flow at end-inspiration.	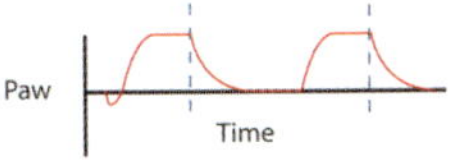

Pressure Support Ventilation Similar to PV (above), with the following differences:	
1) Ppeak is usually lower (unless PSmax is set) 2) Every breath is an assisted breath 3) I to E is flow-cycled (hence T_I may vary between breaths)	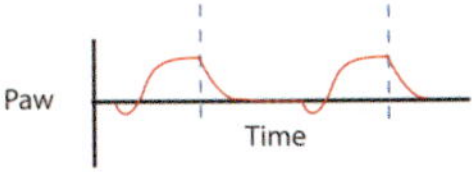

Scalars: Volume-Time

Spontaneous Ventilation

The volume achieved is dependent on patient effort, C, and Raw. The rise to achieved volume is generally sinusoidal.

I to E is patient-cycled

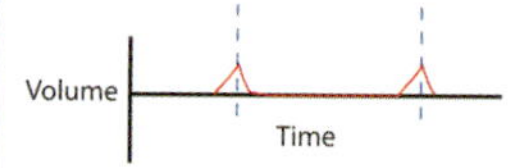

Volume Ventilation – Assist/ Control (constant or square flow)

The volume delivered is determined by the set volume.

The rise to delivered V_T is linear. 1st breath is assisted (patient-triggered). 2nd breath is controlled (machine-triggered).

I to E is volume-cycled.

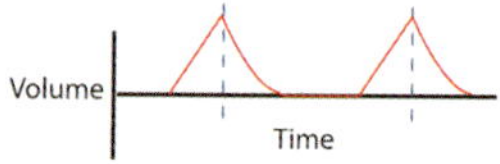

Volume Ventilation – Assist/ Control (decelerating flow)

Same as square flow (above), except that the rise to delivered V_T is usually convex.

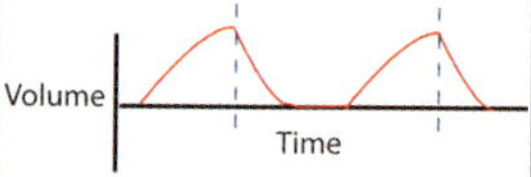

SIMV (constant or square flow)

A combination of assisted VV and spontaneous ventilation.

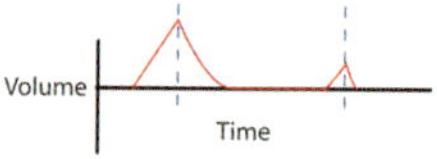

Pressure Ventilation – Assist/ Control The volume delivered is determined by the set pressure level, C, and Raw of the lungs. The rise to deliver the V_T is generally initially rapid, followed by a decrease, and finally a plateau. 1st breath is assisted (patient-triggered). 2nd breath is controlled (machine-triggered). I to E is time-cycled (hence T_I is constant).	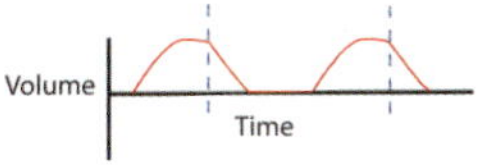

Pressure Support Ventilation Similar to PV (above), with the following differences: 1) The delivered volume (plateau) is usually lower (unless PSmax is set) 2) The delivered volume is dependent on: a) Set pressure support level b) Patient effort, C, and Raw 3) Every breath is an assisted breath 4) I to E is flow-cycled (hence T_I may vary between breaths)	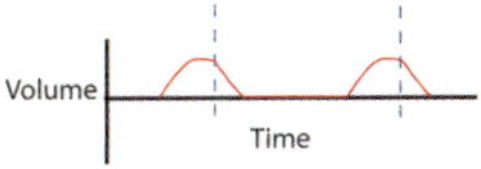

Scalars: Flow-Time

Spontaneous Ventilation The inspiratory curve is usually sinusoidal in shape, but highly variable, depending on patient effort. Peak flows are generally much lower than with ventilator breaths. I to E is patient-cycled	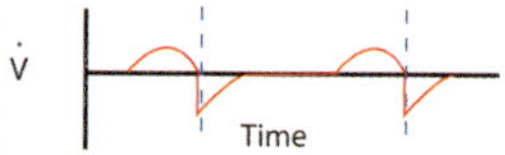
Volume Ventilation – Assist/ Control (constant or square flow) Flow reaches a maximum at the beginning of I and continues at that maximum during the entire inspiratory phase. 1st breath is assisted (patient-triggered). 2nd breath is controlled (machine-triggered). I to E is volume-cycled.	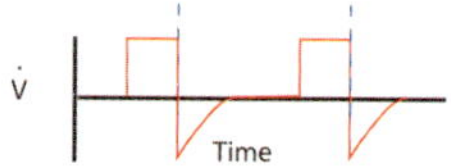
Volume Ventilation – Assist/ Control (decelerating flow) Same as square flow (above), except that inspiratory flow decelerates during the inspiratory phase. Since I to E is volume-cycled, flow may or may not reach zero before end-inspiration.	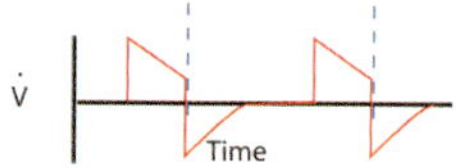
SIMV (square flow) A combination of assisted VV and spontaneous ventilation.	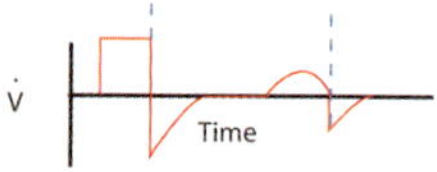

Pressure Ventilation – Assist/ Control

Inspiratory flow reaches a maximum at the beginning of I and then decelerates during the inspiratory phase. Flow is variable depending on patient's C and Raw. 1st breath is assisted (patient-triggered). 2nd breath is controlled (machine-triggered).

I to E is time-cycled (hence T_I is constant). Since I to E is time-cycled, flow may or may not reach zero before end-inspiration. If flow does not reach zero, T_I may be too short.

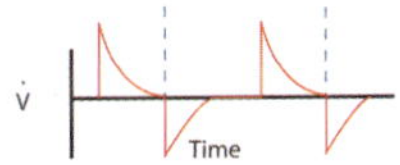

Pressure Support Ventilation

Inspiratory flow reaches a maximum at the beginning of I and then decelerates during the inspiratory phase. Flow is variable depending on patient's C and Raw. Every breath is an assisted breath. I to E is flow-cycled (hence T_I may vary between breaths). I terminates when $\dot{V}_I$ decreases to a ventilator determined flow (usually 25% of peak flow) (flow never reaches zero)

Clinical note: the Flow-Time waveform is the best way to identify a PS breath.

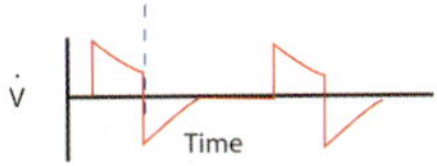

Loops: Pressure-Volume

Spontaneous Ventilation

The loop is clockwise in spontaneous breathing. The inspiratory curve is generally to the left of baseline pressure (vertical axis) due to negative pressure during inspiration. (Negative if ZEEP, less positive if CPAP). The expiratory curve is generally to the right of the baseline pressure due to positive expiratory pressure. The area to the left of the vertical axis represents patient inspiratory WOB (inspiratory resistance). The area to the right of the vertical axis represents patient expiratory WOB (expiratory resistance).

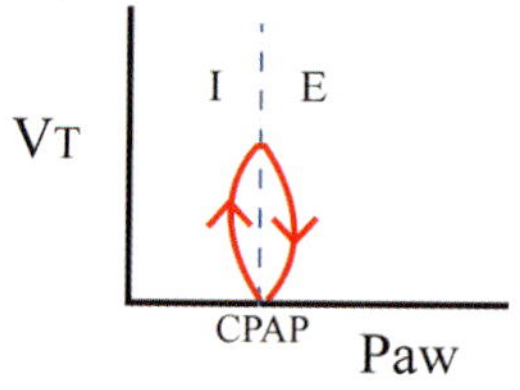

Volume Ventilation – Assist/ Control (constant or square flow)

The loop is counter-clockwise in positive pressure ventilation.

1st breath is assisted (patient-triggered). 2nd breath is controlled (machine-triggered).

During an assisted breath, the inspiratory area to the left of the vertical axis represents the patient WOB required to initiate inspiration. The greater the area, the greater the WOB imposed by the ventilator. Flow-by virtually eliminates imposed WOB. (See enlargement)

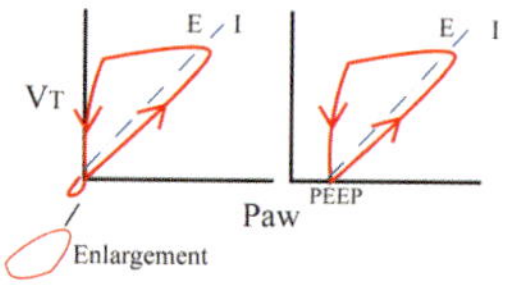

Volume Ventilation – Assist/ Control (decelerating flow)

Same as square flow (above), except the inspiratory limb is more convex.

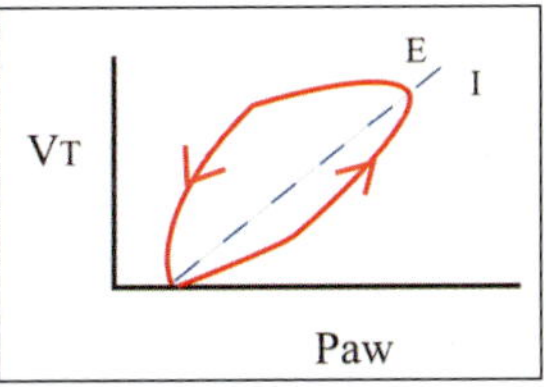

SIMV (constant or square flow)

A combination of spontaneous ventilation and assisted VV.

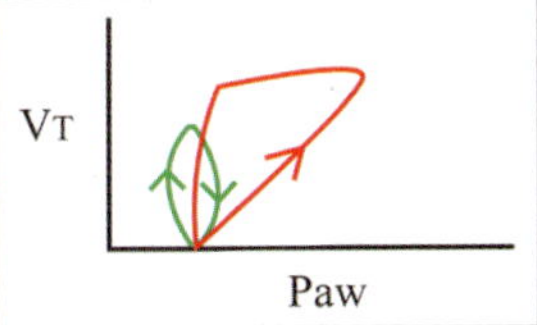

Pressure Ventilation – Assist/ Control

The set pressure is reached quickly before the volume has a chance to rise.

1st breath is assisted (patient-triggered).

2nd breath is controlled (machine-triggered).

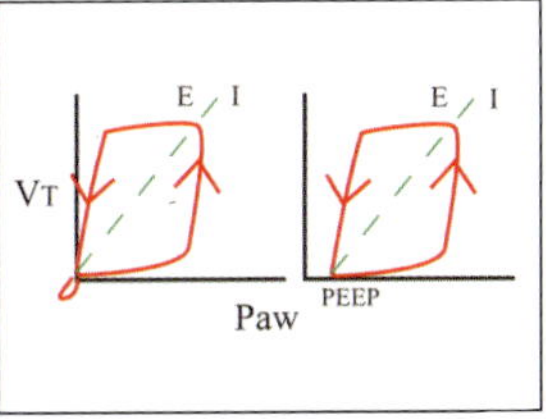

Pressure Support Ventilation

Similar to PV, except:

1) Pressure and volume are usually less (unless PSmax).
2) Each breath is assisted.

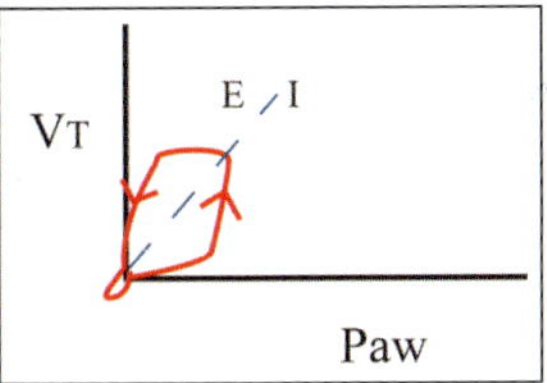

Loops: Flow-Volume

Spontaneous Ventilation
The loop is usually quite circular due to the natural sinusoidal flow rates.

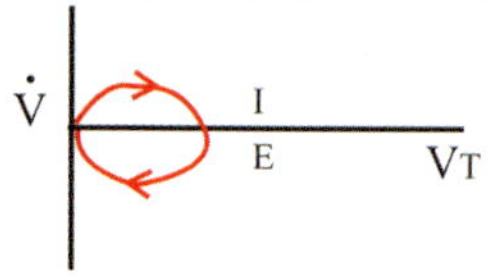

Volume Ventilation – Assist/ Control (constant or square flow)
Flow reaches a maximum at the beginning of I and continues at that maximum during the entire inspiratory phase. V_T is peaked as the flow switches from positive to negative (I to E).

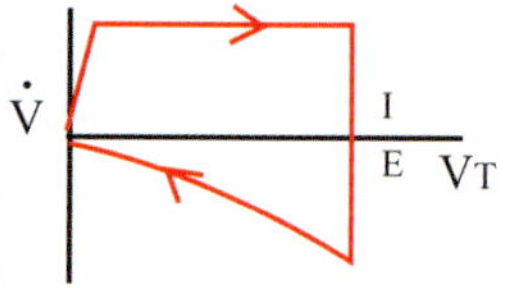

Volume Ventilation – Assist/ Control (decelerating flow)
Same as square flow (above), except inspiratory flow decelerates during the inspiratory phase.

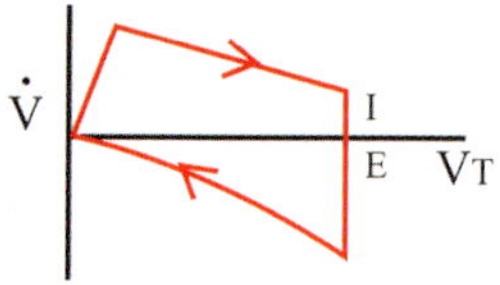

SIMV (constant or square flow)
A combination of spontaneous ventilation and assisted VV.

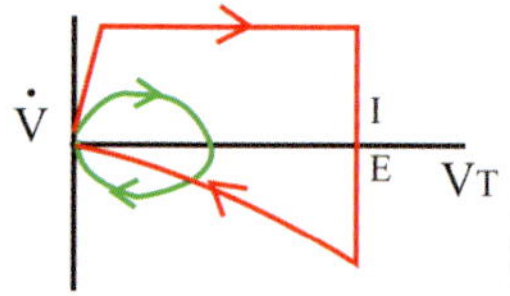

Pressure Ventilation – Assist/ Control Flow reaches a maximum at the beginning of I and then decelerates during the inspiratory phase. V_T is peaked as the flow switches from positive to negative (I to E).	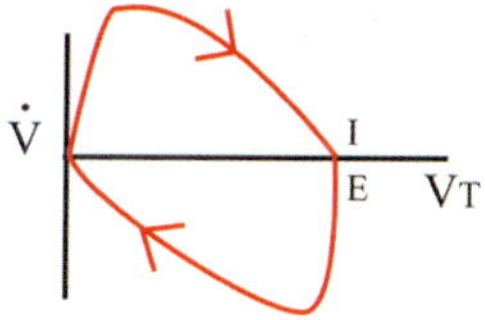
Pressure Support Ventilation Similar to PV, except: 1) Flow and volume are usually less (unless PSmax) 2) The inspiratory phase is terminated when $\dot{V}_I$ decreases to a ventilator determined flow (usually 25% of peak flow) (never reaches zero). 3) Each breath is assisted.	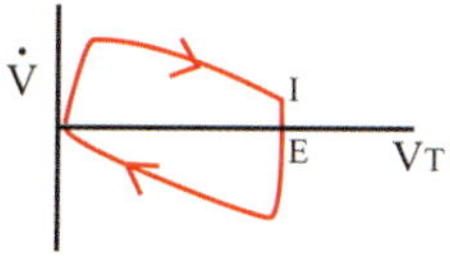

Abnormal Graphic Waveforms by Waveform Type

*** For the description of a particular graph, turn to the Abnormal Graphic Waveform By Problem section and proceed to the particular problem.

All examples are in Volume Ventilation.

Scalars

- Pressure-Time
- Volume-Time
- Flow-Time

Loops

- Volume-Pressure
- Flow-Volume

Abnormal Scalars: Pressure-Time

Air-trapping (auto-PEEP)

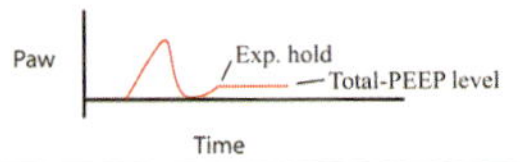

Airway Resistance Changes

↑ PIP-P_{plat}
(5 to 10 cmH_2O)
(Dashed line depicts Pplat)

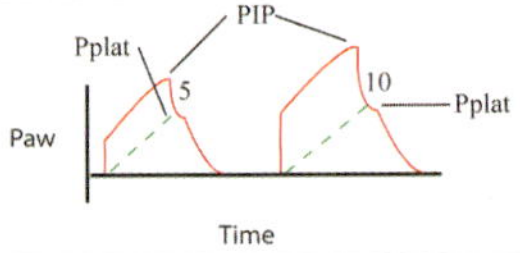

Compliance Changes

↑Pplat
Raw remains the same at 5 cmH_2O
(Dashed line depicts Pplat)

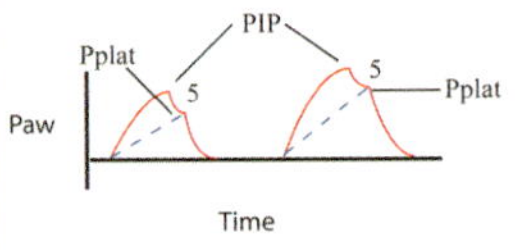

Leaks

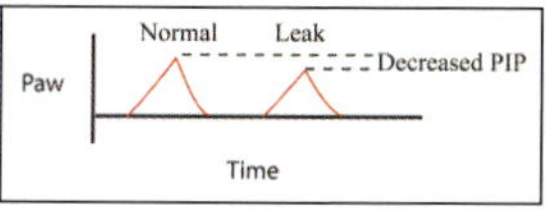

Rate (Cycle) Asynchrony

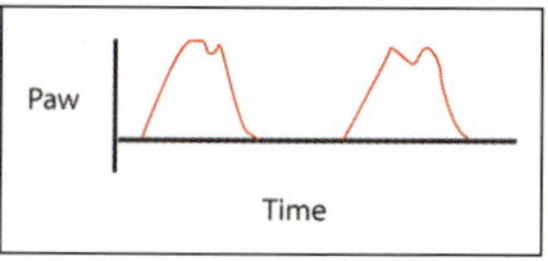

Flow Asynchrony (Flow Starvation) in Volume Ventilation

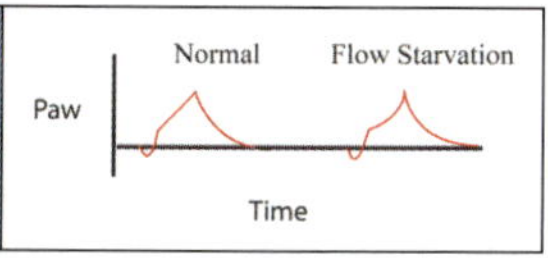

Trigger Asynchrony (Inappropriate Sensitivity Setting)
(Mimics auto-PEEP triggering asynchrony)

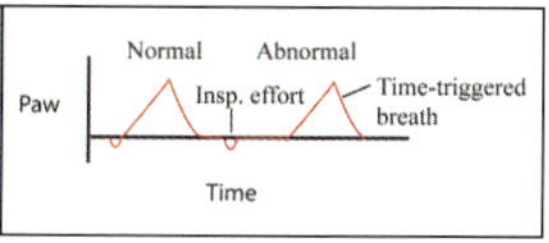

Trigger Asynchrony (Auto-PEEP)

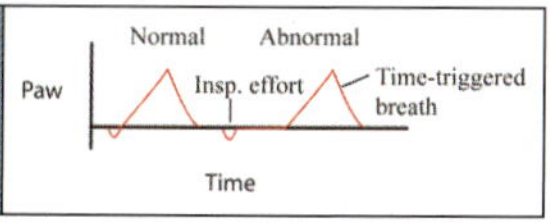

Abnormal Scalars: Volume-Time

Air-trapping (auto-PEEP) Can mimic a leak (see below)

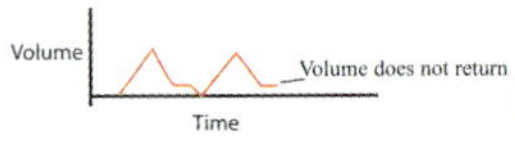

Airway Resistance Changes

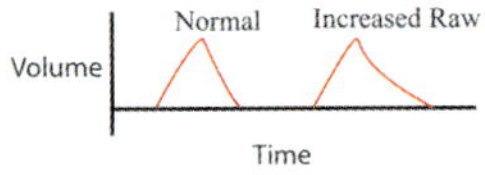

Excessive (Active) Exhalation

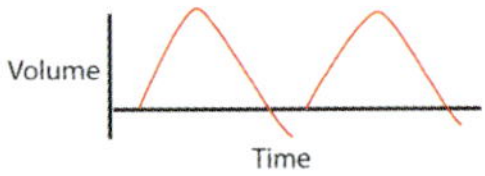

Leaks

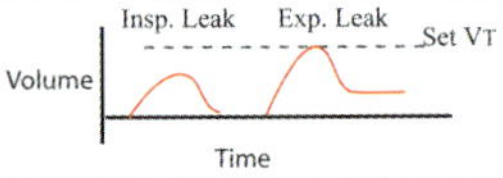

Abnormal Scalars: Flow-Time

Air-trapping (auto-PEEP)

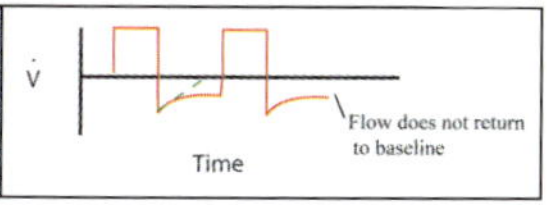

Airway Resistance Changes

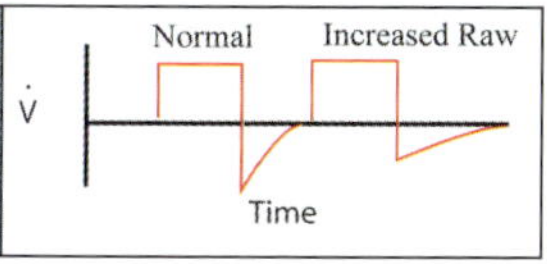

Partial Obstruction

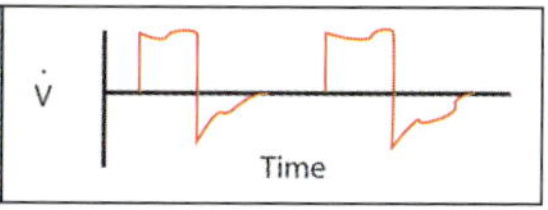

Leaks

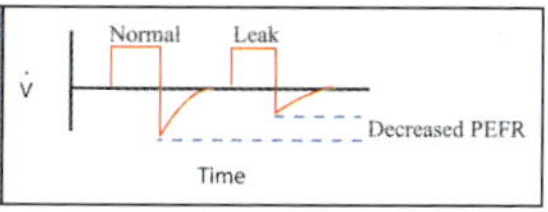

Rate (Cycle) Asynchrony

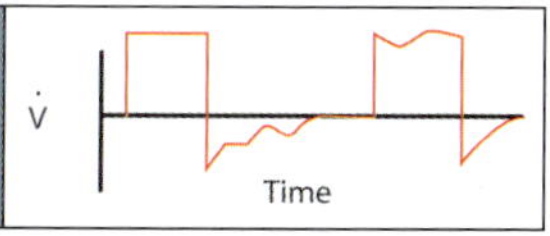

Trigger Asynchrony (Inappropriate Sensitivity Setting)

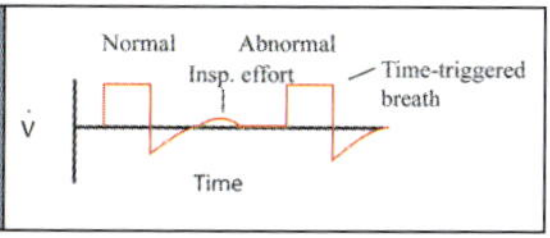

Trigger Asynchrony (Auto-PEEP)

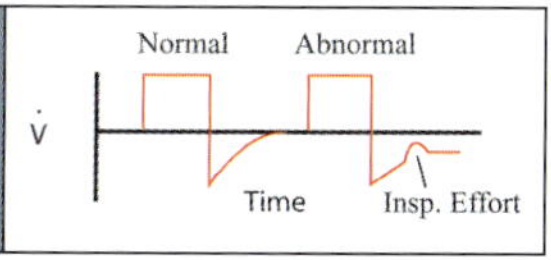

Abnormal Loops: Volume-Pressure

Air-trapping (auto-PEEP)
Example: Volume Ventilation

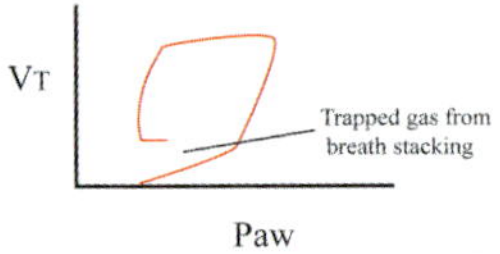

Airway Resistance Changes (Mechanical Breath)
Dashed lines depicts normal and solid line is ↑ Raw
Example: Volume Ventilation

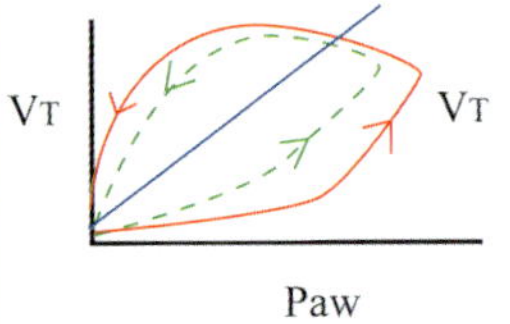

Airway Resistance Changes (Spontaneous Breath)
Dashed lines depicts normal and solid line is ↑ Raw

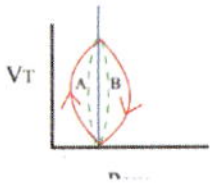

Compliance Changes Example: Volume Ventilation

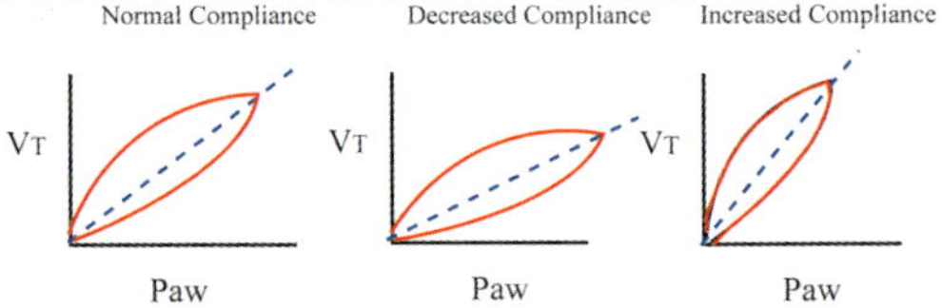

Excessive (Active) Exhalation
Example: Volume Ventilation

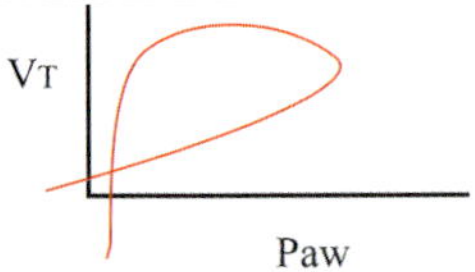

Partial Obstruction

Example: Volume Ventilation

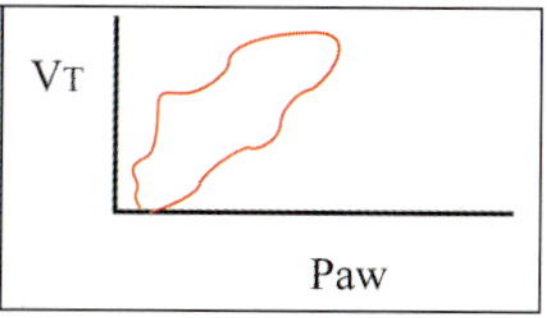

Over-distension

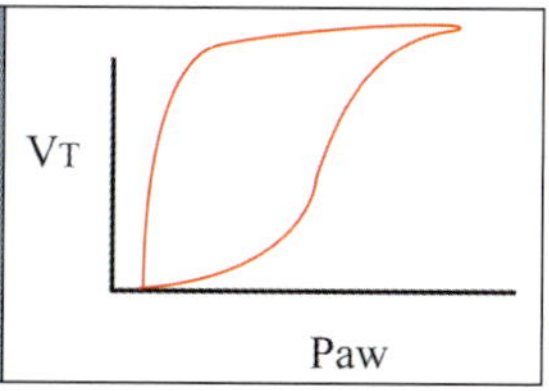

Leaks

Example: Volume Ventilation

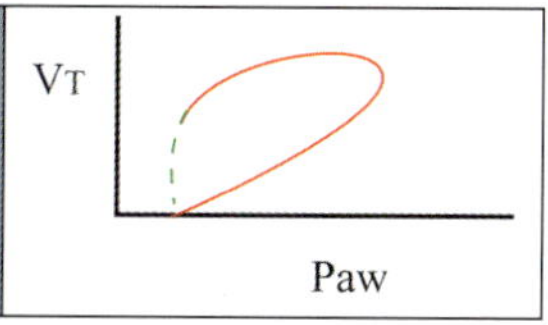

Rate (Cycle) Asynchrony

Example: Volume Ventilation

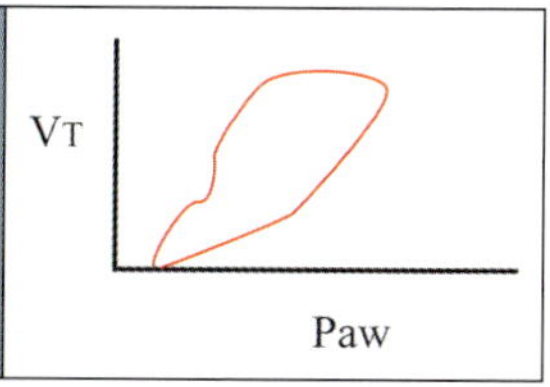

Flow Asynchrony (Flow Starvation)

Example: Volume Ventilation

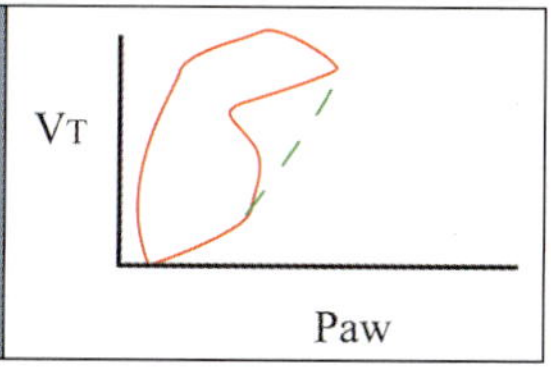

Trigger Asynchrony (Inappropriate Sensitivity Setting)

Example: Volume Ventilation

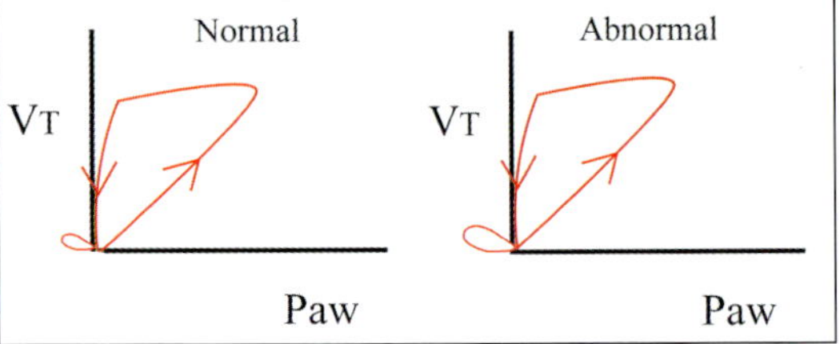

Abnormal Loops: Flow-Volume

All examples are Volume Ventilation

Air-trapping (auto-PEEP)

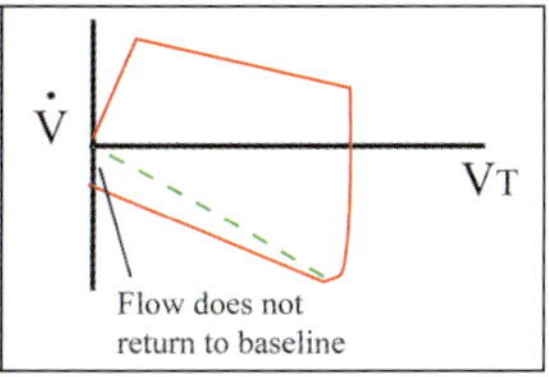

Airway Resistance Changes

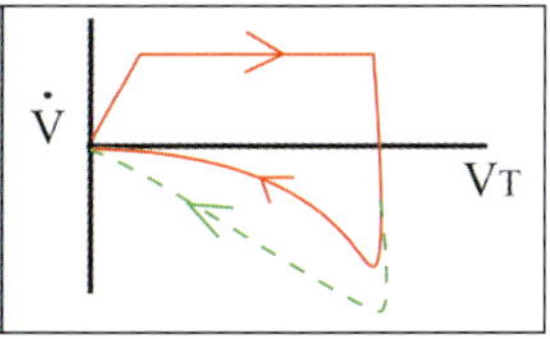

Excessive (Active) Exhalation

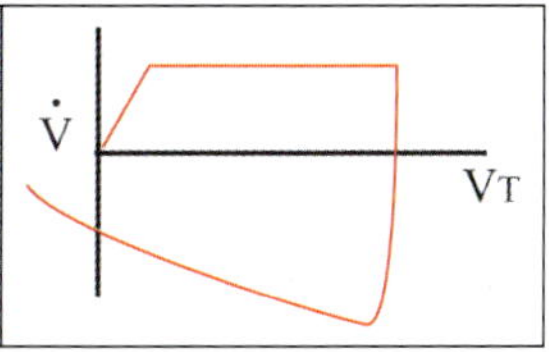

Partial Obstruction

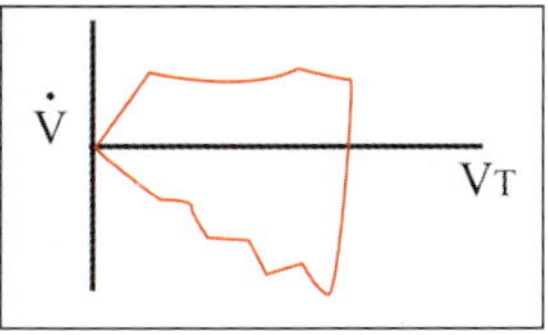

Leaks

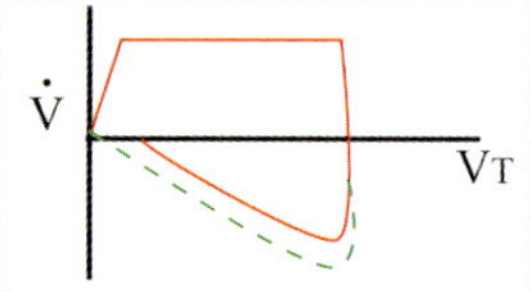

Rate (Cycle) Asynchrony

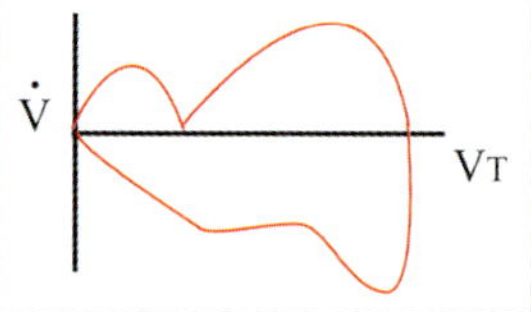

Abnormal Graphic Waveforms by Problem

Section Contents

Patient

- Air-trapping (auto-PEEP)
- Airway resistance changes
- Compliance changes
- Excessive exhalation
- Partial obstruction

Ventilator

- Over-distension
- Leaks

Patient-Ventilator Interaction

- Rate asynchrony
- Flow asynchrony
- Trigger asynchrony (inappropriate sensitivity setting)
- Trigger asynchrony (auto-PEEP)

All examples are in Volume Ventilation.

PATIENT

Air Trapping (auto-PEEP)

Possible Causes

Dynamic hyperinflation (insufficient T_E for complete expiration) due to:

1) Increased expiratory Raw (prolonged expiration)
2) Decreased T_E (insufficient time before next breath)

Early collapse of unstable alveoli during expiration (exhaled air is blocked from flowing out)

Auto-PEEP: Scalars

Pressure-Time

Auto-PEEP can only be identified (and quantified) when an expiratory hold is employed. During the hold, baseline pressure line rises to the auto-PEEP level (depicting pressure still trapped in alveoli). If applied PEEP is employed, the expiratory hold baseline will rise to total PEEP (applied PEEP + auto-PEEP).

Clinical Note: Sufficient hold time must be employed to allow the pressure to reach a plateau, plus there must be not patient respiratory effort during the hold.

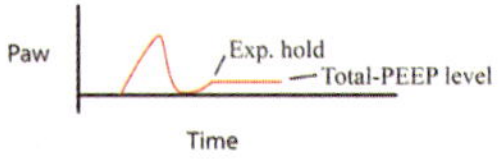

Volume-Time

Volume does not return to baseline (depicting volume still trapped in alveoli). The less the return, the greater the air-trapping. *Note:* this is the same curve as a leak –see Leak.

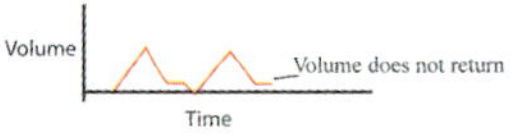

Flow-Time

Expiratory flow does not return to baseline (depicting flow still trapped in alveoli). The less the return, the greater the air-trapping. The dashed line depicts normal flow return to baseline.

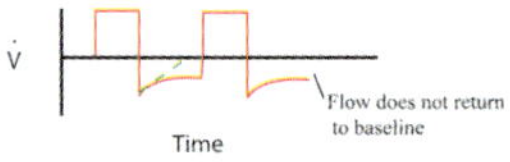

Auto-PEEP: Loops

Volume-Pressure Volume does not return to baseline (depicting volume still trapped in alveoli). The less the return, the greater the air-trapping.	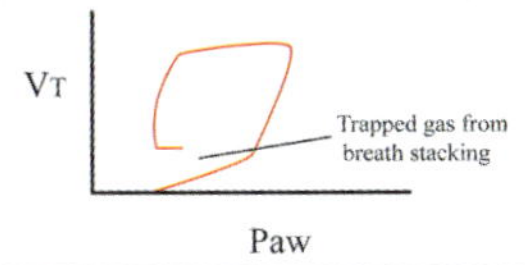
Flow-Volume Expiratory flow does not return to baseline (depicting flow still trapped in alveoli). The less the return, the greater the air-trapping. The dashed line depicts normal flow return to baseline.	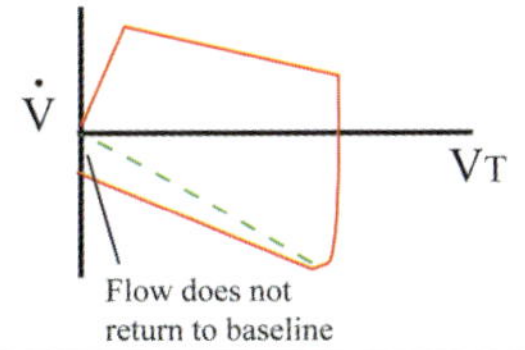

Airway Resistance Changes:

Possible Causes

- Bronchospasm
- Damp or blocked expiratory filter
- ET tube (small size, bitten, kinked, or partially obstructed)
- High $\dot{V}$I
- Secretion buildup (see also water/secretion problem)

Descriptions:
All examples are Volume Ventilation

Raw Δ: Scalars

Pressure-Time
Using an inspiratory pause (hold), the difference between Ppeak and Pplat can be visualized and measured.
1st waveform: Ppeak – Pplat = 5 cmH_2O
2nd waveform: Ppeak – Pplat = 10 cmH_2O
Clinical Notes: An increased Ppeak while Plat remains the same is indicative of an increased Raw. The reverse situation, a decreased Ppeak while Pplat remains the same, is indicative of a decreased Raw (e.g., a positive bronchodilator response). See Compliance Changes, next section.

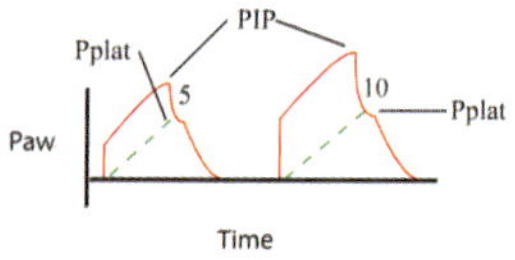

Volume-Time
The time for volume emptying is prolonged with increased Raw

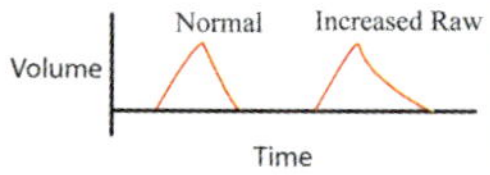

Flow-Time A: normal B: ↑ Raw (expiratory): 1) Peak expiratory flow is decreased 2) Expiratory flow is decreased (flatter slope) 3) Time of expiration is prolonged *Clinical Notes*: Bronchodilator response is determined by the degree to which the increased Raw waveform returns to a normal shape. Inspiratory Raw is generally not well depicted on a flow-time scalar because ventilator-driving force is usually sufficient to overcome it.	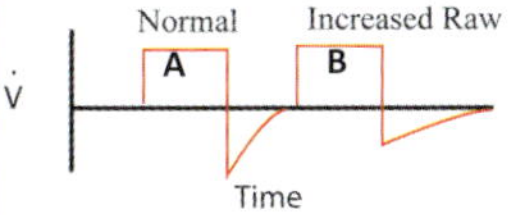

Raw Δ: Loops

Volume-Pressure (mechanical breath) The dashed line depicts a normal loop. The solid line depicts increased Raw. The movement of the upward inspiratory slope to the right is indicative of inspiratory resistance. The movement of the downward expiratory slope to the left is indicative of expiratory resistance.	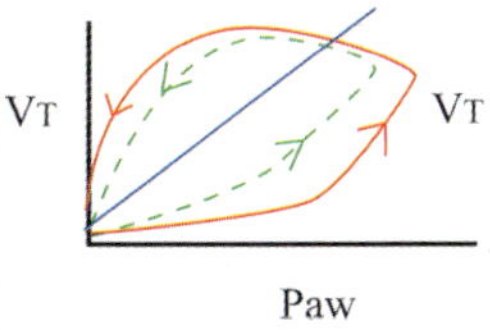

Waveform Graphics

Volume-Pressure (spontaneous breath) The inspiratory area (A) to the left of the vertical baseline will increase with increased inspiratory Raw. The expiratory area (B) to the right of the vertical baseline will increase with an increase in expiratory Raw.	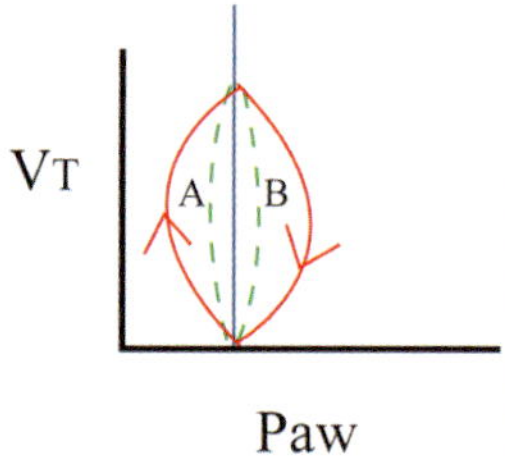

Flow-Volume The dashed line depicts a normal loop. The solid line depicts increased Raw: 1) Decreased peak expiratory flow 2) Concave mid-expiratory flow curve (theoretically due to resistance in medium and small airways. No concavity suggests the resistance is in the large upper airways). 3) V_T may be reduced in some instances *Clinical Notes*: Bronchodilator response is determined by the degree to which the increased Raw waveform returns to a normal shape. Inspiratory Raw is generally not well depicted on a flow-volume loop because ventilator-driving force is usually sufficient to overcome it.	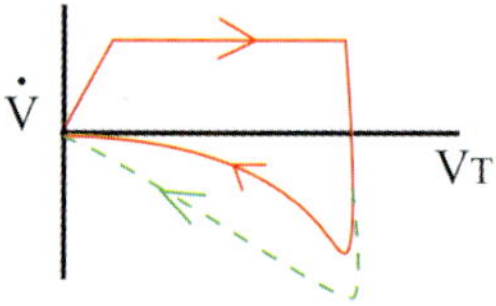

Compliance Changes:

Possible Causes

↓ Compliance (C)	↑ Compliance (C)
• ARDS • Atelectasis • Abdominal distention • CHF • Consolidation • Fibrosis • Hyperinflation • Pleural effusion • Right mainstem intubation • Tension pneumothorax	• Emphysema • Surfactant therapy

Descriptions:
All examples are Volume Ventilation

Compliance Δ: Scalars

Pressure-Time (VV)

Using an inspiratory pause (hold), the difference between Ppeak and Pplat can be visualized and measured.

A: Ppeak – Pplat = 5 cmH_2O

B: Ppeak – Pplat = 5 cmH_2O

Clinical Notes:

If Ppeak and Pplat ↑ along with the Raw (Ppeak-Pplat), this is indicative of ↓ C and ↑ Raw.

See airway resistance changes, previous section. Pressure curves remain unchanged in PV. An ↑ Ppeak plus a similar ↑ in Pplat is indicative of ↓ compliance.

The reverse situation, a ↓ Ppeak plus a similar ↓ in Pplat is indicative of an ↑ compliance.

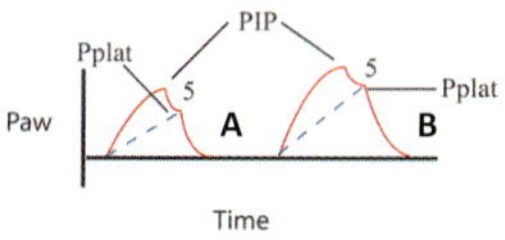

Compliance Δ: Loops

Volume-Pressure

Decreasing compliance: the slope of the imaginary line through the center of the loop moves towards the pressure axis

Increasing compliance: the slope of the imaginary line through the center of the loop moves towards the volume axis.

Clinical Note: Depending on the parameters and scaling, normal compliance curves are conventionally displayed as having a 45° slope

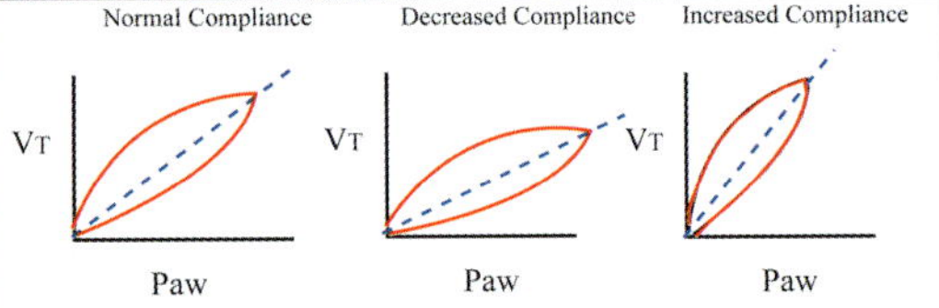

Excessive (Active) Exhalation:

Possible Causes

- Patient is exhaling below FRC due to:
- Air-trapping (excessive exhalation occurs periodically in an attempt to relieve the trapped volume).
- Pain
- Positional change

Note: a consistent, regular pattern of excessive exhalation indicates an equipment calibration problem.

Descriptions:

Excessive (Active) Exhalation: Scalars

Volume-Time

Volume curve dips below zero baseline

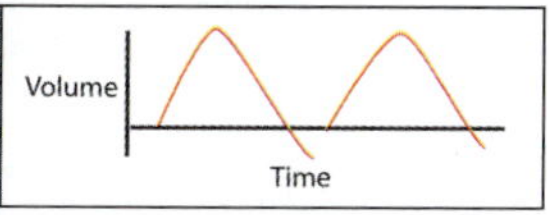

Excessive (Active) Exhalation: Loops

Volume-Pressure

Expiration curve continues below the zero volume point.

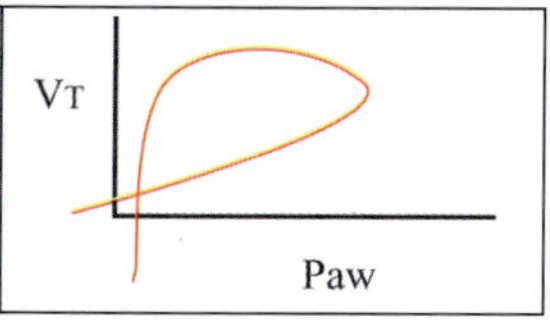

Flow-Volume

Expiration curve continues to the left of the zero volume point.

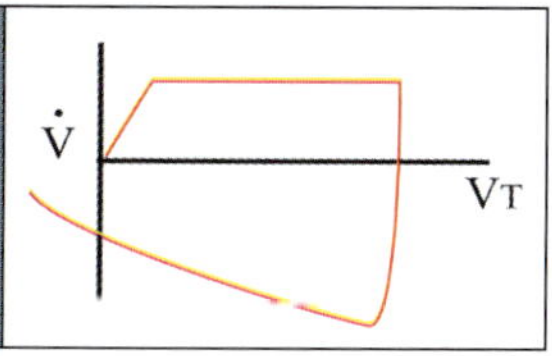

Partial Obstruction:

Possible Causes

- Indwelling suction catheter left partially in ET tube
- Flap of tissue, Mucous plug
- Water/secretions in airways/circuit

Descriptions:

Partial Obstruction: Scalars

Flow-Time
The obstruction is moved by flow moving in and out of the airways/circuit resulting in fluctuating flow.

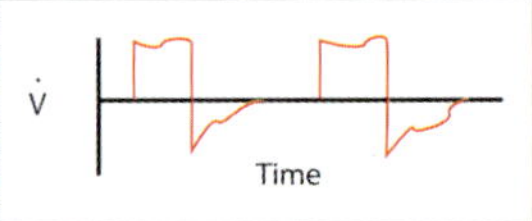

Partial Obstruction: Loops

Volume-Pressure
The obstruction is moved by the flow moving in and out of the airways/circuit, resulting in fluctuating pressure.

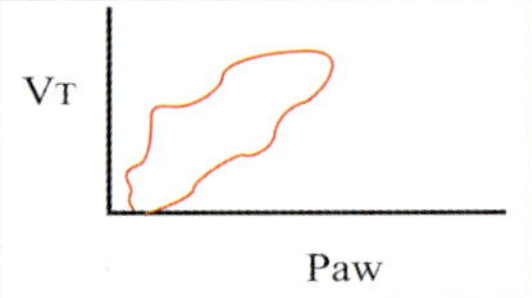

Flow-Volume
The obstruction is moved by the flow moving in and out of the airways/circuit, resulting in fluctuating flow. It will have a "saw tooth" appearance if the obstruction is secretions or water.

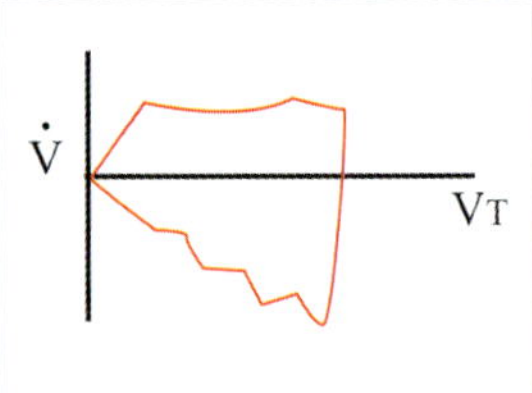

VENTILATOR

Clinical Note: The static V-P loop is the most accurate way of detecting low and high inflection points. Dynamic loops such as the ones depicted in this book do not quantify these points.

Over-distension

Possible Causes

Too much V_T in Volume Ventilation

Too much pressure in Pressure Ventilation

Description:

Volume-Pressure Loop Increasing volume increases pressure for a very little or no increase V_T causing a "Beaking" at end inspiration. (Example in Volume ventilation) Clinical note: "Beaking" doesn't necessarily indicate overdistention; it may be due to patient-ventilator asynchrony.	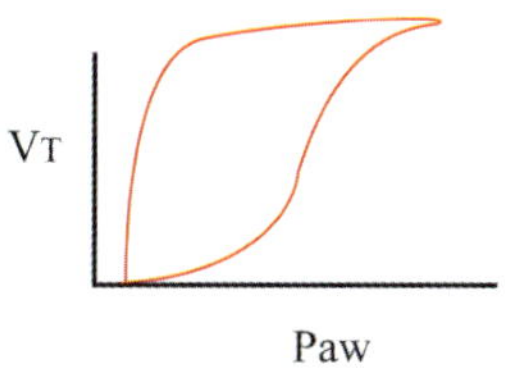

Leaks

Possible Causes

Expiratory	Inspiratory
Air leak through chest tube	Loose connections
BP fistula	Ventilator malfunction
ET tube cuff leak	Faulty flow sensor
NG tube in trachea	

Clinical Note: Leaks are generally expiratory. Set volumes will not be reached if the leak is inspiratory. A leak in the circuit between the ventilator and flow transducer would result in a smaller volume (both I and E); pressure and flow are then set by the ventilator. A volume loss around neonatal cuffless tubes is normal. Lost volume should not exceed 20% of total volume.

Leaks: Scalars

Pressure-Time

Ppeak will be ↓ (esp. VV) due to ↓ returned volume and/or an inspiratory leak.

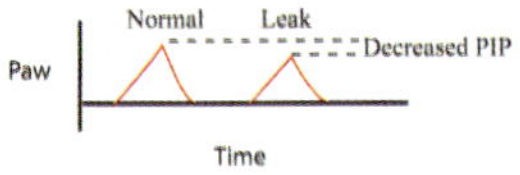

Volume-Time

Set volume is not reached with an inspiratory leak. The returned volume does not return to baseline with an expiratory leak.

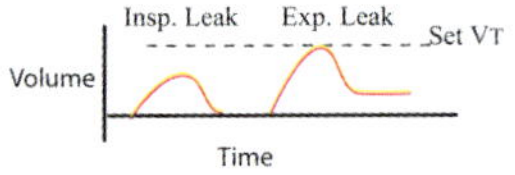

Flow-Time

Peak expiratory flow is ↓ due to ↓ returned volume.

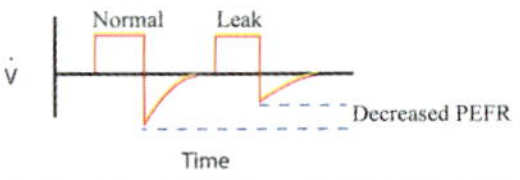

Leaks: Loops

Volume-Pressure Volume does not return to zero baseline, resulting in an incomplete loop. The dashed line depicts a loop without a leak.	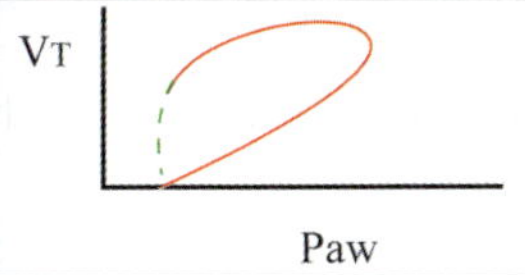
Flow-Volume Volume does not return to zero baseline, resulting in an incomplete loop. The dashed line depicts a loop without a leak.	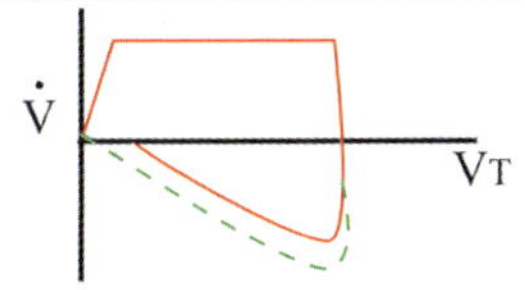

Rate (Cycle) Asynchrony:

Possible Causes

- Neurological injury
- Patient air-hunger

Descriptions:

Rate (Cycle) Asynchrony: Scalars

Pressure-Time
Erratic inspiratory and/or expiratory phases indicate inspiratory and/or expiratory efforts to inhale or exhale.

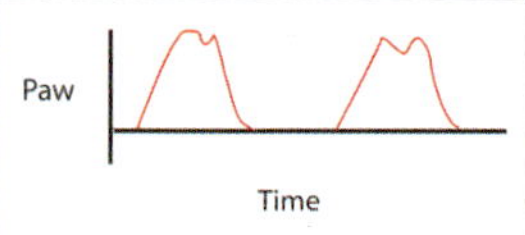

Flow-Time
Erratic inspiratory and/or expiratory phases indicate inspiratory and/or expiratory efforts to inhale or exhale.

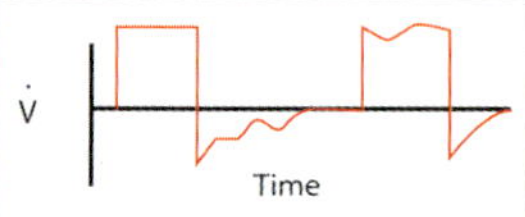

Rate (Cycle) Asynchrony: Loops

Volume-Pressure
Erratic inspiratory and/or expiratory phases indicate inspiratory and/or expiratory efforts to inhale or exhale.

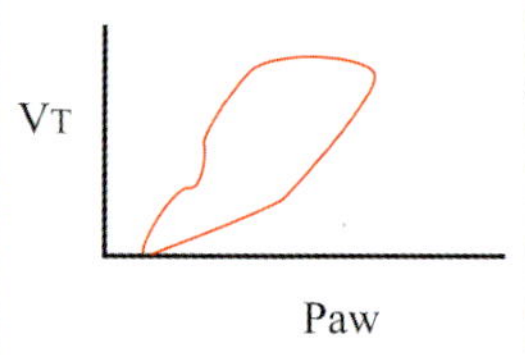

Flow-Volume
Erratic inspiratory and/or expiratory phases indicate inspiratory and/or expiratory efforts to inhale or exhale.

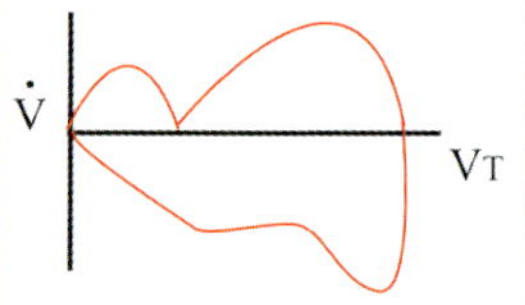

Flow Asynchrony (Flow Starvation)

Descriptions:

Flow Asynchrony (Flow Starvation): Scalars

Pressure-Time
The inspiratory limb is concave with a negative pressure deflection due to the patient's attempt to pull more flow. The expiratory curve will be unaffected by flow starvation.

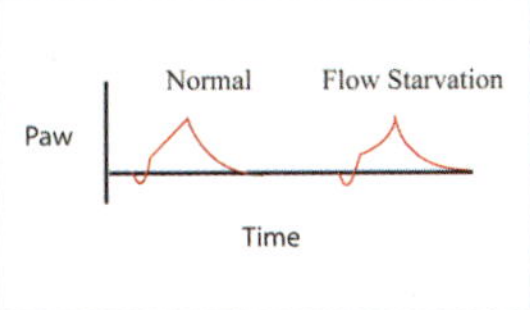

Clinical Note: Adjusting Peak Flow rate:
In VV, the rate of rise in pressure (upward slope) is related to the peak flow setting. An inadequate flow presents as a slow and often concave rise to peak pressure. A high flow will present as a very fast rise to peak pressure (mimicking PV).

Flow Asynchrony (Flow Starvation): Loops

Volume-Pressure
The inspiratory limb is concave with a negative pressure deflection due to the patient's attempt to pull more flow. The expiratory curve will be unaffected by flow starvation

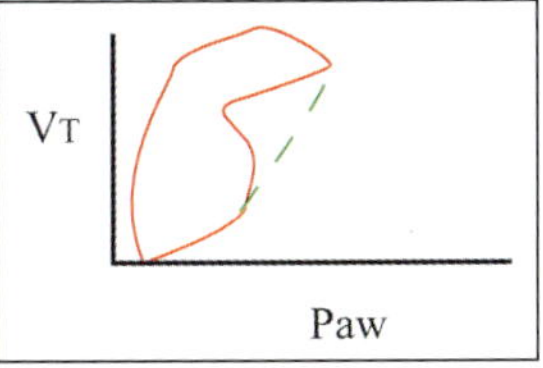

Trigger Asynchrony (Inappropriate Sensitivity Setting)

Descriptions:

Trigger Asynchrony (Sensitivity): Scalars

Pressure-Time
Negative inspiratory pressure is applied by the patient, however it is not enough to trigger a machine breath.

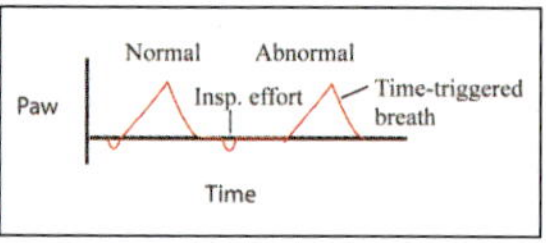

Flow-Time
As the patient attempts to trigger the ventilator, the flow turns slightly positive then negative due to a futile effort.

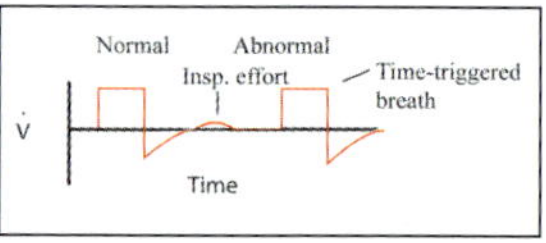

Trigger Asynchrony (Sensitivity): Loops

Pressure-Volume
Normal – the negative deflection is minimal.
Abnormal – the negative deflection is greater. The greater the negative deflection, the greater the effort to trigger.

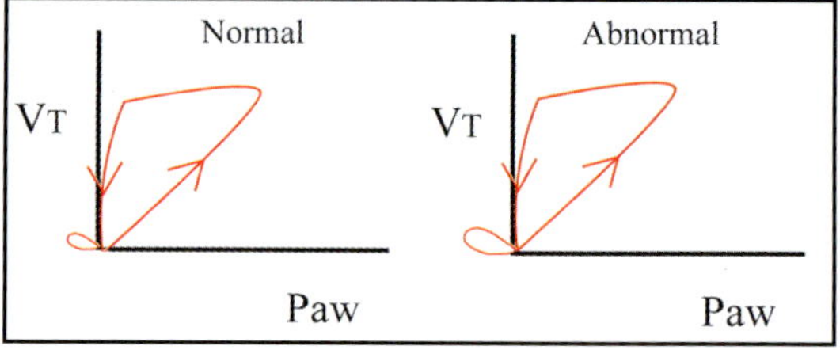

Trigger Asynchrony (Auto-PEEP)

Descriptions:

Trigger Asynchrony (Auto-PEEP): Scalars

Pressure-Time

Normal – the negative deflection is minimal.

Abnormal – the neg. deflection is greater. The greater the negative deflection, the greater the effort to trigger. There is no difference in this graph compared to the "Inappropriate Sensitivity Setting" Pressure-Time Scalar.

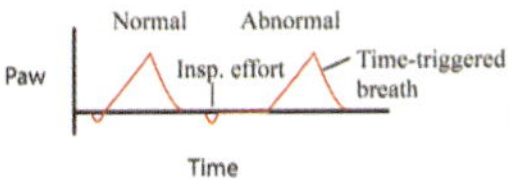

Flow-Time

As the patient attempts to trigger the ventilator, the expiratory flow curve turns slightly positive then negative due to a futile effort. The difference between this graph and the "Inappropriate Sensitivity Setting" Flow-Time Scalar is that the flow turns + within auto-PEEP area below baseline.

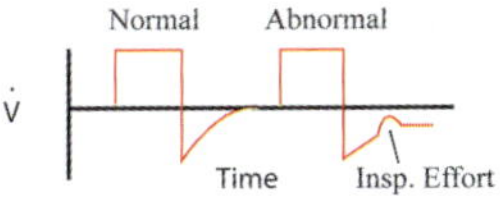

Clinical Note: Inappropriate setting and auto-PEEP trigger asynchrony could be combined.

Other Applications

Pressure-Time Scalars

Determining machine breath types (VV) Negative pressure deflection just prior to inspiration indicates an assisted breath.	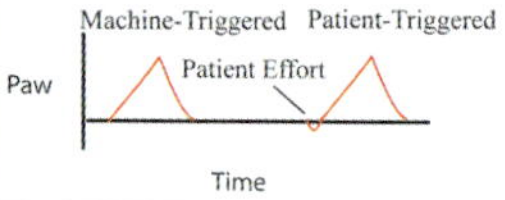
Assessing plateau pressure In VV, an inspiratory pause will cause the breath pressure to plateau. The clinician can then separate resistance from compliance to determine the cause of an increase/decrease in Ppeak. • Raw ~ Ppeak – Pplat • Crs ~ Pplat – PEEP See Chapter 7 for Equations to calculate *Clinical Note*: In PV, Ppeak = Pplat, provided zero flow at end-inspiration.	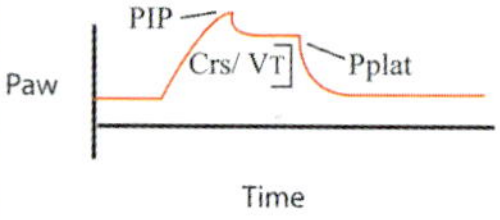

Setting rise-to-pressure time in PV (controlled or supported) The faster the flow, the quicker set pressure is reached in the I phase. This is used in conjunction with the flow-time scalar (see next section). A rise-to-pressure time too fast could cause a spike or "ringing" in the airways and cause the patient to become asynchronous.	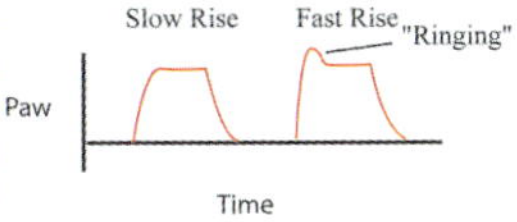

Switching cycling criteria and optimizing inspiratory phase in a pressure support breath. Ventilators have specific flow-cycling criteria for pressure-supported breaths. Some ventilators have backup pressure and time-cycling features that can be adjusted (depending on the ventilator). In the example shown, the first breath is pressure-cycled. Note the pressure spike at the end of inspiration, indicating that the flow-cycling parameter (e.g., 25%) is too low and that the patient is attempting to exhale. Adjusting the expiratory sensitivity or the time-cycling parameter, the clinician can limit the inspiratory phase, which should improve patient comfort.	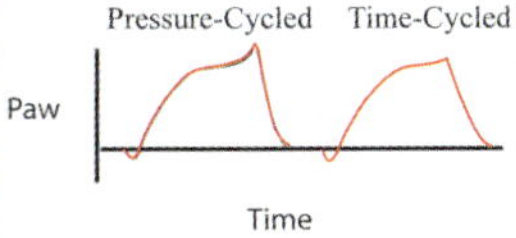

Flow-Time Scalars

Verifying waveform shapes
Some ventilators have flow waveform options in VV. The flow-time scalar is used to verify the waveform selected.

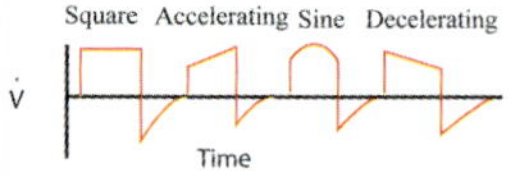

Setting I-time in PV
When lengthening or shortening the inspiratory time, the flow-time scalar should be used to see if there is more flow available for additional volume delivery. Once the V̇I has reached zero (baseline), there will be no volume ↑ with an ↑ I-time (except slight increases due to long TCs).

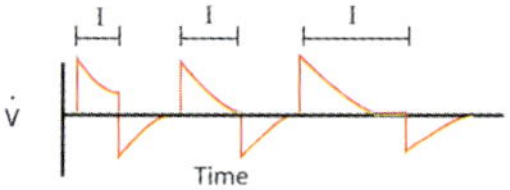

Setting rise-to-pressure time in PV (controlled or supported)
The faster the flow, the quicker set pressure is reached in the I phase. This is used in conjunction with the P-T scalar (see previous section).

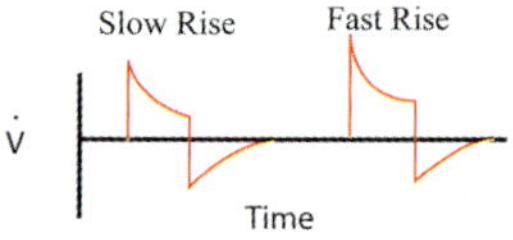

Volume-Pressure Loop

Assessing inspiratory effort
The clockwise loops below the baseline pressure depict patient inspiratory effort in assist ventilation.

- A (red): increased (inappropriate) trigger effort
- B (green): minimum (appropriate) trigger effort

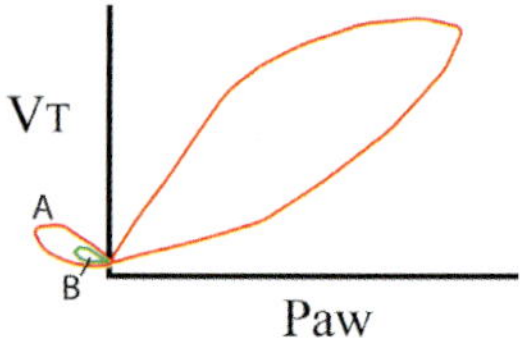

Make It Your Own

Notes Page

Make It Your Own

Notes Page

7 Equations

CONTENTS

Acid-Base 7-2
Oxygenation 7-4
Ventilation 7-10
Ventilator Calculations 7-14
Mechanics 7-14
Weaning 7-21
Perfusion/Hemodynamics 7-22
Patient Calculations 7-26
Miscellaneous 7-27

These are the major categories within this chapter. Equations are listed alphabetically within each section.

Equation	Comments	Significance
Acid-Base		
Anion Gap 1) $AG = Na^+ - (Cl^- + HCO_3)$ 2) $AG = (Na^+ + K^+) - (Cl^- + HCO_3)$	Normal = 12 (± 4) mEq/L Normal = 20 (± 4) mEq/L AG = the difference between measured cations (+) and anions (–) (ie., unmeasured ions)	Indicates metabolic acidosis due to an increase of acid (rather than a decrease of base) ↑ AG = ↑ unmeasured anions (acid): ↑ **acid production**: lactate (hypoxia), ketones (diabetes) ↑**acid addition**: poisons (methanol, salicylates) ↓ **acid excretion**: renal failure ↓ **AG** = ↓ unmeasured anions: albumin
Note: When an Anion Gap Metabolic Acidosis is present, there are various methods used to calculate for additional or mixed metabolic disorders. See Oakes' ***ABG Pocket Guide: Interpretation and Managemen***t for more details.		
Base Excess (BE) 1) $BE = \frac{\Delta PaCO_2 + \Delta pH \times 100}{2}$ 2) $BE \approx \Delta PaCO_2$ 3) $BE \approx \Delta HCO_3 + 10\ \Delta pH$	$\Delta PaCO_2$ from 40 ΔpH from 7.40 ΔHCO_3 from 24	Base deficit (BD) = - BE Accurate only in ranges of: $PaCO_2$ 30-50, pH 7.30-7.50

Equation	Comments	Significance
Bicarbonate Correction of pH HCO_3 = (0.2)body weight x BD	Corrects to pH 7.40 BD = base deficit	Used to correct for metabolic acidosis.
Henderson-Hasselbach 1) $pH = 6.1 + \log HCO_3/ H_2CO_3]$ 2) $pH = 6.1 + \log [HCO_3/\text{dissolved } CO_2]$ 3) $pH = 6.1 + \frac{\text{total } CO_2 - 0.03PaCO_2}{0.03PaCO_2}$ 4) $PaCO_2 = \frac{\text{total } CO_2}{0.3 \times [1 - \text{antilog}(pH - 6.1)]}$	Total $CO_2 = \frac{\text{volume \%}}{2.2}$	Calculation of pH or $PaCO_2$.
Rule of 8's At: pH — HCO_3 = 7.6 — 8/8 ($PaCO_2$) 7.5 — 6/8 ($PaCO_2$) 7.4 — 5/8 ($PaCO_2$) 7.3 — 4/8 ($PaCO_2$) 7.2 — 3/8 ($PaCO_2$)	Examples: when pH 7.4, $PaCO_2$ 40, HCO_3 = 5/8 (40) = 25 pH 7.3, $PaCO_2$ 60, HCO_3 = 4/8 (60) = 30	Estimate of HCO_3 in relation to pH and $PaCO_2$.

Equation	Comments	Significance
T40 Bicarbonate $T40 = HCO_3 - \text{expected } \Delta HCO_3$	HCO_3 = standard plasma Expected $\Delta HCO_3 = \frac{PaCO_2 - 40}{15}$	Used to find a "true" metabolic component in acute hypercapnia.
Winters Formula $PaCO_2$ predicted $= 1.54 \times HCO_3 + 8.36 (\pm 1)$	Measures respiratory compensation for metabolic acidosis.	$PaCO_2$ (actual) > $PaCO_2$ (pred) = mixed acidosis $PaCO_2$ (actual) < $PaCO_2$ (predicted) = respiratory alkalosis
Oxygenation		
A-a Gradient ($PA\text{-}aO_2$) ($A\text{-}aDO_2$) Alveolar- arterial O_2 tension difference 1) $PA\text{-}aO_2 = PAO_2 - PaO_2$	Normal = 10 - 25 mm Hg (air) = 30 - 50mm Hg (100% O_2) Increases with age and FIO_2. PaO_2 is calculated at FIO_2 0.5 breathed x 20 min to get PaO_2 > 150 (100% not used due to ↑ shunt).	Indicates efficiency of gas exchange. Normal values indicate normal shunt. Distinguishes between true shunt and V/Q mismatch. ↑ = shunt, V/Q mismatch, alveolar hypoventilation, or ↓ diffusion. > 350 mm Hg indicative of weaning failure.
2) $PA\text{-}aO_2 = 140 - (PaO_2 + PaCO_2)$	ABG is drawn for $PaCO_2$ and PaO_2.	Less accurate estimate (on 21% only).
3) $PA\text{-}aO_2 / 20$	Estimate of shunt (100% O_2)	See shunt equation.

Equation	Comments	Significance
Alveolar O_2 Tension (Alveolar air equation) (PAO_2) 1) P_AO_2 = ([PB - PH_2O] x FIO_2) – $PaCO_2$ x (FIO_2 + 1 - FIO_2/RE)	Normal =100 mm Hg(air) = 663 mm Hg (100%, sea level) RE = respiratory exchange ratio (normal = 0.8)	Partial pressure of O_2 in alveoli. Used to determine alveolar O_2 tension to calculate PA-aO_2 gradient, a/A ratio, and % shunt.
2) P_AO_2 = ([PB - PH_2O] x FIO_2) – $PaCO_2$ (1.25)	Short form when breathing < 100% O_2	
3) P_AO_2 = PIO_2 - $PaCO_2$ (1.25)	Short form when breathing 100% O_2. PIO_2 = (PB - PH_2O) x FIO_2	
4) P_AO_2 = 150 - $PaCO_2$ (1.25)	Estimate only on room air	
5) P_AO_2 = (FIO_2 x 700) - 50	Estimate only	
Arterial/Alveolar O_2 Tension (a/A Ratio) PaO_2 / P_AO_2	Index of gas exchange function or efficiency of the lungs. Normal = 0.8 - 0.9 (0.75 elderly) at any FIO_2.	More stable than A-a gradient: A-a gradient changes with FIO_2, a/A remains relatively stable with FIO_2 changes. Changes only with $PaCO_2$ or V/Q changes. Low a/A (<0.6) = shunt, V/Q mismatch, or diffusion defect; < 0.35 indicative of weaning failure, <0.15 = refractory hypoxemia.
PaO_2 known / P_AO_2 calculated = PaO_2 desired / P_AO_2 unknown	Useful to predict PaO_2 when changing FIO_2 (See FIO_2 estimation equation)	Can be used to estimate shunt (See shunt equation).

Equation	Comments	Significance
Arterial-(mixed)Venous O_2 Content Difference ($Ca\text{-}\bar{v}O_2$) $CaO_2 - C\bar{v}O_2 = Ca\text{-}\bar{v}O_2$	Difference between arterial and mixed venous O_2 contents. Normal = 4.2 - 5.0 mL/dL (vol%)	Represents O_2 consumption by tissue and estimate of cardiac output. ↑ = ↓CO or ↑ metabolism. ↓ = ↑CO or ↓ metabolism.
Arterial-(mixed)Venous O_2 Tension Difference ($Pa\text{-}\bar{v}O_2$ or $a\text{-}\bar{v}DO_2$) $PaO_2 - P\bar{v}O_2 = Pa\text{-}\bar{v}O_2$	Normal = 60 mm Hg	Difference between arterial and mixed venous O_2 tensions.
Arterial CO_2 tension ($PaCO_2$) **PaCO2** = $\frac{\dot{V}CO_2}{\dot{V}A}$	Normal = 35-45 mm Hg	
FIO2 Estimation 1) Using a/A ratio: $PAO_2 = PaO_2$ desired / a/A ratio	Figured at any FIO_2.	Used to estimate the FIO_2 needed to achieve a desired PaO_2 or the PaO_2 that will be achieved at any given FIO_2.
2)Using alveolar O_2 tension: $FIO_2 = PAO_2 + (PaCO_2 / 0.8) / (PB\text{–}H_2O)$	Need ↑ FIO_2 x 20 minutes	$\frac{\text{Current } PaO_2}{\text{Current } FIO_2} = \frac{\text{Desired } PaO_2}{\text{New } FIO_2}$
3)Using A-a gradient: $FIO_2 = PA\text{-}aO_2$ + desired PaO_2 / 760		
4) Using P/F Ratio: PaO_2 should be: $\frac{5\ PaO_2}{1\ FIO_2}$		New $FIO_2 = PaO_2$ desired + $PaCO_2$ desired / (PaO_2 / PAO_2) / $(PB - H_2O)$
5) Estimate: $FIO_2 = PaO_2 / 500$		

Equation	Comments	Significance
O_2 Consumption (Demand) ($\dot{V}O_2$) $\dot{V}O_2 = CO \times (CaO_2 - C\bar{v}O_2) \times 10$ $= CO \times Ca\text{-}\bar{v}O_2 \times 10$	Normal = 200 - 250 mL/min	Volume of O_2 consumed (utilized) by the body tissues per min. Index of metabolic level and CO. $\uparrow\dot{V}O_2$ = ↑metabolism or CO; $\downarrow\dot{V}O_2$ = ↓metabolism or CO
O_2 Consumption Index ($\dot{V}O_2I$) $\dot{V}O_2I = CI \times Ca\text{-}\bar{v}O_2 \times 10$	$\dot{V}O_2I = \dot{V}O_2/BSA$ $= 110\text{-}165\ mL/min/m^2$	O_2 consumption per body size.
O_2 Content 1) Arterial $CaO_2 = (Hgb \times 1.36) \times SaO_2 + (PaO_2 \times 0.0031)$ 2) Venous (mixed) $C\bar{v}O_2 = (Hgb \times 1.36) \times S\bar{v}O_2 + (P\bar{v}O_2 \times 0.0031)$ $= \dot{V}O_2/CO$ 3) Pulmonary capillary CcO_2	Normal = 15-24 mL/dL (vol%) Both 1.36 and 1.39 are considered correct. Hgb = gm % Normal = 12-15 mL/dL (vol%) $P\bar{v}O_2$ = pressure in mixed venous blood obtained from pulmonary artery. See shunt equation.	Total amount of O_2 in arterial blood (combined plus dissolved). Total amount of O_2 in mixed venous blood (combined plus dissolved). SaO_2 and $S\bar{v}O_2$ obtained from oximeter or oxyheme dissociation curve.

Equation	Comments	Significance
O_2 Delivery (Supply, Transport) ($\dot{D}O_2$) $\dot{D}O_2 = CO \times CaO_2 \times 10$	Normal = 750-1000 mL/min Quantity of O_2 delivered to the body tissues per minute. Requires CO determination.	$\uparrow O_2$ transport $= \uparrow CO$ +/or $\uparrow CaO_2$ $\downarrow O_2$ transport $= \downarrow CO$ +/or $\downarrow CaO_2$ 10 = conversion factor to mL/min
O_2 Delivery Index ($\dot{D}O_2I$) $\dot{D}O_2I = CI \times CaO_2 \times 10$	$\dot{D}O_2I = \dot{D}O_2$ / BSA = 500-600 mL/min/m^2	O_2 delivery per body size.
O_2 Extraction Ratio (O_2 ER) $O_2\ ER = \frac{O_2 \text{ consumption (demand)}}{O_2 \text{ delivery (supply)}}$ $= \frac{\dot{V}O_2}{\dot{D}O_2} \times 100$ $= \frac{Ca\text{-}\bar{v}O_2}{CaO_2}$	Normal = 25 % Amount of O_2 extracted and consumed by the body tissues, relative to the amount delivered. Estimate $= \frac{Sa\text{-}\bar{v}O_2}{SaO_2}$	Indicator of O_2 supply/demand balance. $\uparrow$ratio = $\downarrow O_2$ +/or $\uparrow O_2$ transport $\downarrow$ ratio = $\uparrow O_2$ +/or $\downarrow O_2$ transport
O_2 Index (OI)	$OI = (\overline{P}aw \times FIO_2 \times 100) / PaO_2$	> 40 = severe respiratory distress with high mortality; 20 - 25 = mortality > 50%
O_2 Reserve O_2 Reserve $= \dot{D}O_2 - \dot{V}O_2$	Normal = 750 mL/min $= CO \times C\bar{v}O_2 \times 10$	Venous O_2 supply: O_2 supply minus O_2 demand

Equation	Comments	Significance
O2 Saturation (mixed venous) ($S\bar{v}O_2$) $S\bar{v}O_2 = SaO_2 - \dot{V}O_2/\dot{D}O_2$ $= SaO_2 - Sa\text{-}\bar{v}O_2$	Normal = 75 % (60-80 %)	Percent of hemoglobin in mixed venous blood, saturated with O_2.
P/F Ratio (Oxygenation Ratio) PaO_2 / FIO_2	Normal = 400 – 500 (regardless of FIO_2) What PaO_2 Should Be: $\frac{5\ PaO_2}{1\ FIO_2\%}$	< 300 indicative of ALI < 200 = ARDS
Predicted PaO_2 (based on age)	$PaO_2 = 110 - \frac{1}{2}$ age	
Respiratory Index (RI) $PA\text{-}aO_2 / PaO_2$	Normal = < 1.0	1.0- 5.0 = V/Q mismatch > 5.0 = refractory hypoxemia due to physiol. shunt
Respiratory Quotient (Exchange ratio) (RQ, RE, RR) 1) $RQ = \frac{\dot{V}CO_2}{\dot{V}O_2}$ 2) $RQ = \dot{V}E \times \frac{F\bar{E}\ CO_2 - F_ICO_2}{F_IO_2 - F\bar{E}\ O_2}$ 3) $RQ = \frac{F\bar{E}\ CO_2}{FIO2 - F\bar{E}\ O_2}$	$\frac{\text{Volume } CO_2 \text{ produced/min}}{\text{Volume } O_2 \text{ consumed/min}}$ Normal = 200 / 250 = 0.8	RQ = ratio of CO_2 produced to O_2 consumed (internal respiration). RE represents the amount of O_2/CO_2 exchange in the lungs per minute (external respiration). RE = RQ in steady state condition.

Equation	Comments	Significance
Ventilation/Perfusion Index (VQI) $VQI = \frac{1 - SaO_2}{1 - S\bar{v}O_2}$	Normal = 0.8	Combines assessment of SaO_2 and $S\bar{v}O_2$ to estimate venous admixture. Correlates well with $\dot{Q}_S/\dot{Q}_T$.
Ventilation		
Alveolar Ventilation ($\dot{V}_A$) 1) $\dot{V}_A = \dot{V}_E - \dot{V}_D$ 2) $\dot{V}_A = (V_T - V_Dphys) \times f$ 3) $\dot{V}_A = (\dot{V}_ECO_2/PaCO_2) \times 863$ 4) Ideal $\dot{V}_A = (\dot{V}_ECO_2/ PaCO_2$ desired) x 863 5) $\dot{V}_A \times PaCO_2$ known $= \dot{V}_A \times PaCO_2$ desired	Normal = 4 - 6 L/min $\dot{V}_ECO_2 = \dot{V}_E$ measured x $F\bar{E}\ CO_2$ calculated or measured $F\bar{E}\ CO_2 = P\bar{E}\ CO_2$ measured / $P_B - PH_2O$ 863 = correction factor if in milliliters, (0.863 = if in liters). Estimated $\dot{V}_ECO_2$ = 3mL/kg/min	The volume of inspired air which participates in gas exchange per minute. Used to calculate the ideal alveolar ventilation needed to maintain a desired $PaCO_2$.
Alveolar Volume (V_A) 1) $V_A = \dot{V}_A / f$ 2) $V_A = V_T - V_D$ 3) $V_A = 2 \times$ IBW (lbs) 4) $V_A = 2/3\ V_T$	 Estimate Estimate (normal)	The volume of each breath that participates in gas exchange.

Equation	Comments	Significance
Deadspace Ventilation ($\dot{V}_D$) 1) $\dot{V}_Dphys = V_Dphys \times f$ 2) $\dot{V}_Dphys = \dot{V}_E - \dot{V}_A$ 3) $\dot{V}_Dphys = (PaCO_2 - PECO_2 / PaCO_2) \times \dot{V}_E$ 4) $\dot{V}_Dphys = \dot{V}_D/V_T \times \dot{V}_E$	Normal = 1/3 $\dot{V}_E$	The volume of wasted air (not participating in gas exchange) per minute.
Deadspace Volume (V_D) 1) $V_D = V_T - V_A$ 2) $V_D = \dot{V}_E - \dot{V}_A / f$ 3) $V_Dphys = V_Danat + V_Dalv + V_Dmech + V_Dcomp$ = total V_D	Normal = 1/3 V_T V_Danat = anatomical V_D (1 mL/lb IBW; 0.5 mL/lb with ET tube or trach) V_Dalv = alveolar V_D V_Dmech = mechanical (10mL/inch) VDcomp = tubing compliance loss	The volume of wasted air (not participating in gas exchange) per breath (V > Q). ↑V_Dalv = ↓ CO, pulmonary vasoconstriction, pulmonary embolus

Equation	Comments	Significance
Deadspace / Tidal Volume Ratio (V_D/V_T Ratio) 1) Bohr Equation: $\frac{V_D phys}{V_T} = \frac{PaCO_2 - P\bar{E}CO_2}{P_ACO_2}$ $\frac{V_D anat}{V_T} = \frac{PetCO_2 - P\bar{E}CO_2}{PetCO_2}$	Normal = 0.33 $\frac{(150\ V_D)}{(450\ V_T)}$ $P\bar{E}CO_2$ = mixed expired Normal = 0.33 (no ABG required) Pet = end tidal	Used to measure the portion of V_T not participating in gas exchange (wasted ventilation). $V_D/V_T > 0.5$ is indicative of respiratory failure. Many lung diseases (atelectasis, pneumonia, pulmonary edema, emboli, etc.) can exhibit changes in V_D (i.e., $V_D alv$) without corresponding changes in $PaCO_2$.
2) Estimate: $V_D phys / V_T = (\dot{V}_E$ actual / $\dot{V}_E$ predicted) x ($PaCO_2$ actual / 40) x 0.33	This equation is quite accurate. No mixed expired sample required.	
Minute Ventilation ($\dot{V}_E$) (Minute Volume) 1) $\dot{V}_E = V_T \times f$ 2) $\dot{V}_E = \dot{V}_A + \dot{V}_D$ 3) $\dot{V}_E \approx 1/PaCO_2$ 4) New $\dot{V}_E = \dot{V}_E$ current x $PaCO_2$ current/ $PaCO_2$ desired 5) $PaCO_2$ desired x $\dot{V}_E$ needed = $PaCO_2$ current x $\dot{V}E$ current 6) Nomogram (See next page)	Normal = 5 - 7 L/min. Changing f is often preferred to changing V_T (due to altering V_D/V_T ratio). $\dot{V}_A$ = effective alveolar ventilation $\dot{V}_D$ = physiological deadspace	The total air in or out of the lungs in one minute. Used to calculate the $\dot{V}_E$ needed to maintain a desired $PaCO_2$. Change rate to change $\dot{V}_E$, changing V_T may alter the V_D/V_T ratio.

Equation	Comments	Significance
Ventilation/Perfusion Ratio ($\dot{V}/\dot{Q}$ Ratio) $\dot{V}_A/\dot{Q}c = \frac{(C\bar{v}CO_2 - CaCO_2) \times 8.63}{PaCO_2}$	Normal = $\frac{4L/min}{5L/min}$ = 0.8 Ratio of minute alveolar ventilation to minute capillary blood flow. Represents external respiration.	Ratio changes represent the degree and type of respiratory imbalances. ↓ Ratio (↓V/Q) = atelectasis, COPD, pneumonia, pneumothorax, N-M disorders, etc. ↑ Ratio (V/↑Q) = shock, pulmonary emboli, cor pulmonale, PPV.

Nomogram to estimate minute ventilation required to maintain a given PaCO2 when VD/VT is known:
To obtain the require minute ventilation to achieve a given PaCO2, the minute ventilation is plotted against the PaCO2 (measured simultaneously) and the VD/VT ratio is read on the isopleth that corresponds to the intersection. The isopleth is then followed to the desired PaCO2 and the corresponding minute ventilation read off the vertical axis.

For example: A patient with a VE of 5L and a PaCO2 of 60 mmHg has an estimated VD/VT ratio of 0.40. To achieve a desired PaCO2 of 40 mmHg, follow the 0.40 isopleth up to correspond to the PaCO2 of 40 on the horizontal axis. Then read the appropriate minute ventilation of about 8L/min off the vertical axis.

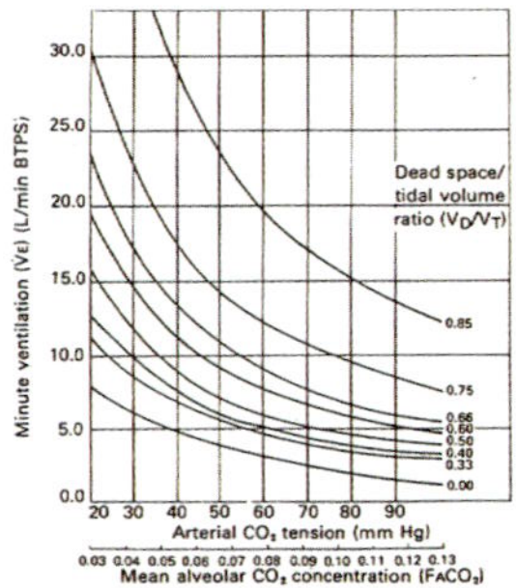

Equation	Comments	Significance
Ventilator Calculations		
Ventilator Flow $\dot{V} = \dot{V}_E \times RFF$ or $\dot{V} = \dot{V}_E \times 1/TI\%$	RFF = ratio flow factor = I + E Example: I:E ratio = 1:3, RFF = 4	Used to calculate proper flow to deliver a V_T in a given T_I.
Ventilator Rate Needed for Desired $PaCO_2$ New rate = $\frac{\text{current rate} \times PaCO_2}{\text{desired } PaCO_2}$	Desired $\dot{V}_E$ = $\frac{\text{present } PaCO_2 \times \text{present } \dot{V}_E}{\text{desired } PaCO_2}$	This equation holds presuming a steady metabolic rate, stable or no spontaneous breathing, and no change in other ventilator parameters, or V_{Dmech}.
Mechanics		
Airway Occlusion Pressure (P0.1)	Normal = < 2 cm H_2O Change in airway pressure at 0.1 sec after beginning inspiration against an occluded airway. Used to assess ventilatory drive and demand. Indicative of ventilatory demand.	↑ P0.1 = ↑ patient workload +/or drive (possible inadequate ventilator support). ↓ P0.1 = ↓ patient workload +/or drive (possible excessive ventilator support). > 4 - 6 cm H_2O is indicative of weaning failure. (See PImax) Although actual value is negative, it is reported as a positive.

Equation	Comments	Significance
Airway Resistance (Raw) 1) $R = \Delta P / \dot{V}$ 2) Raw = Pmouth - Palv / $\dot{V}_I$ 3) Raw = PIP - Pplat / $\dot{V}_I$ 4) Raw = Cdyn - Cstat (see below)	Normal = 0.5 - 2.5 cm H_2O/L/sec @ 0.5 L/sec (30 L/min) ET tube = 4 - 8 cm H_2O/L/sec $\dot{V}_I$ = inspiratory flow in L/sec, square wave flow pattern (use 30 L/min if comparing with norm).	Represents frictional resistance of air-flow (80%) and tissue motion (20%). Raw ≈ $1/r^4$ ↑ airflow resistance = airway collapse, edema, bronchospasm, secretions, ET tube etc. ↑ tissue resistance = pulmonary edema, fibrosis, pneumonia, etc. > 5 cm H_2O/L/sec may = wean failure.
Clinical Note: A quick estimate of Raw: = P_{TA} (transairway pressure) = PIP - Pplat ↑P_{TA} = ↑Raw ↓P_{TA} = ↓Raw	↑PIP + ↑Pplat (P_{TA} constant) = ↓Cstat ↑PIP + same Pplat (↑P_{TA}) = ↑Raw ↓PIP + ↓Pplat (P_{TA} constant) = ↑Cstat ↓PIP + same Pplat (↓P_{TA}) = ↓Raw	Pressure support is used primarily to overcome airway resistance of circuit and ET tube. Appropriate PS level can be estimated as PTA (i.e., PIP - Pplat). Note: By convention Raw refers to inspiratory Raw. Expiratory Raw may be determined by PIP - PEEP / $\dot{V}$expir and is typically > inspiratory Raw.

Equation	Comments	Significance
Compliance (C) $C = \Delta V / \Delta P$ $C_{LT} = C_L + C_{CW}$ $= \Delta V / Palv - PB$ $C_L = \Delta V / Palv - Ppl$ $C_{CW} = \Delta V / Ppl - PB$	Normal = 70 - 100 mL/cm H_2O Total compliance is referred to as C_{LT} (lung + thorax) or Crs (respiratory system). C_L = lung compliance C_{CW} = chest wall (thorax) compliance	Represents the ease of distention of the lungs and thorax. Includes elastic, functional, and tissue viscous resistance. Ideal = 100mL/ cm H_2O Lungs and chest wall each = 200 mL/ cm H_2O. P_B = barometric pressure; Ppl = pleural pressure Palv = alveolar pressure

Equation	Comments	Significance
Static Compliance (Cstat) How To Measure Cstat = V_T - Vtubing / Pplat - PEEP Pplat = the pressure needed to maintain lung inflation during zero airflow. It is measured by using either an inspiratory hold or temporarily occluding the exhalation port until pressure stabilizes (approx 1 - 4 sec). PEEP = PEEPE + PEEPI Clinical Note: In VV, a ↓Cstat results in an ↑PIP and ↑Pplat (V_T constant). In PV, a ↓Cstat results in a ↓V_T (PIP and Pplat constant).	Normal = 70 - 100 mL/cm H_2O Vtubing = volume loss in tubing due to circuit compliance Vtubing = CF (tubing compliance factor) x Pgradient (Pplat - PEEP) CF must be determined for each patient-ventilator setup (normals range from 1.5 - 5.0 mL/cm H_2O). It is either calculated by newer ventilators or manually by: setting V_T to 200 mL, triggering the ventilator, occluding the patient wye, and observing PIP. CF = V_T (200) / PIP (Pplat can be used in place of PIP). V_{tubing} = (V_T (200) / PIP) x (Pplat - PEEP)	Represents the combination of lung elasticity and chest wall recoil. Usually measured while on MV. ↓ Cstat = ↓ lung elasticity or ↓ chest wall recoil. ↑ Cstat = ↑ lung elasticity or ↑ chest wall recoil. Trend changes in Cstat and Cdyn are more significant in interpreting lung conditions than single measurements. A Cstat ≤ 25- 33 mL/cm H_2O is indicative of weaning failure. Cstat can also be used to determine optimal PEEP.

Equation	Comments	Significance
Dynamic Compliance (Cdyn) How To Measure Cdyn = V_T - Vtubing / PIP - PEEP Usually measured while on MV.	Normal = 40 - 70 mL/cm H_2O Vtubing = CF x (PIP - PEEP) (See Cstat above to determine CF) PEEP = $PEEP_E$ + $PEEP_I$	Represents the combination of static lung compliance (Cstat) and airway resistance (Raw). For conditions causing ↑ or ↓Cdyn, see Cstat (above) Trend changes in Cstat and Cdyn are more significant in interpreting lung conditions than single measurements.
Clinical Notes: In VV, a↓Cdyn results in an↑PIP (V_T constant). In VV, a ↓PIP (V_T constant) = improved Cstat or Raw or a leak. In PV, a ↓Cdyn results in a ↓V_T (PIP constant). In PV, an ↑V_T (PIP constant) = improved Cstat or Raw.	↑Cdyn (same Cstat) =↓Raw ↓Cdyn (same Cstat) = ↑Raw ↑Cdyn (with same↑ in Cstat) = ↑Cstat ↓Cdyn (with same ↓ in Cstat) = ↓Cstat ↑Cdyn (with partial ↑ in Cstat) =↓Raw and ↑Cstat ↓Cdyn (with partial ↓ in Cstat) = ↑Raw and ↓Cstat	

Equation	Comments	Significance
Equation of Motion $Pawo = V/C + (Raw \times \dot{V})$	Elastic components of respiratory system: $P = V/C$ $V = P \times C$ $C = V/P$ Resistive components of respiratory system: $P = Raw \times \dot{V}$ $\dot{V} = P/Raw$ $Raw = P/\dot{V}$	At any moment the airway opening pressure (Pawo) must exactly balance the opposing lung and chest wall expansion forces. P, $\dot{V}$I, + V can be controlled by the clinician. In VV: Set $\dot{V}$: P varies with Raw Set V: P varies with C In PV: Set P: $\dot{V}$ varies with Raw Set P: V varies with C
Maximal Inspiratory Pressure (PImax) (MIP, NIP) Two methods: Marini #1- total occlusion @ end-exhalation Marini #2- total occlusion @ below FRC	The maximal inspiratory effort (pressure) generated against an occluded airway (approx 20 sec). Normal < 20 cm H_2O (i.e., < - 20 cm H_2O) Although actual value is negative, it is reported as a positive.	Indicative of the capability of the inspiratory muscles. (See P0.1 above) P0.1 / PImax = demand / capability = predictive weaning index ≤ 0.9 indicative of weaning failure Prior to start of test patient should be actively breathing (remove vent support). Remove $PEEP_E$ and $PEEP_I$. Respiratory muscles should not be fatigued.

Equation	Comments	Significance
Mean Airway Pressure ($\overline{P}aw$) $\overline{P}aw = \frac{(T_I \times PIP) + (T_E \times PEEP)}{Ttot}$ $\overline{P}aw = (PIP - PEEP) \times T_I/Ttot + PEEP$	Average airway pressure during several breathing cycles.	$\overline{P}aw = ([P_{TA} + ½\ PA] - PEEP) \times T_I/Ttot + PEEP$ Note: Should always be less than CVP (1 cm H_2O = 0.735 mmHg)
Rapid - Shallow Breathing Index (RSBI) RSBI = f / V_T or $f^2 / \dot{V}_E$	Measure f and V_T (in liters) while off the ventilator. Normal = < 100	Has proven to be one of the best predictive indices for weaning. > 105 is indicative of weaning failure
Time Constant (TC) TC = Raw x Cstat TC = $\Delta P/\dot{V} \times \Delta V/\Delta P$ Note: TC generally refers to inspiratory TC. Expiratory TC may be much longer than inspiratory TC in COPD.	1TC = 63% 2TC = 87% 3TC = 95% 4TC = 98% 5TC = 99% % = % of V_T entering lungs within each TC period. Normal TC = 0.2 sec Normal T_I = 3 - 4 TC = 3 or 4 x 0.2 sec = 0.6 – 0.8 sec	TC (inspir) indicates alveolar filling time. ↑ TC (> 0.2 sec) is usually indicative of ↑Raw (but may be ↑C_{LT}). ↓ TC (< 0.2 sec) is usually indicative of ↓C_{LT} (but may be ↓Raw). TC(expir) indicates alveolar emptying time. < 3 TCexpir will generally result in air-trapping. TCexpir may be approximated with a F-V loop.

Equation	Comments	Significance
Vital Capacity (VC)	Normal is 60-80 mL/kg	< 60 mL/kg indicates general restr. process > 10 mL/kg is needed for effective deep breathing and cough. < 10 mL/kg = impending respiratory failure
Work of Breathing (WOB) $W = \int P \times V$ WOB / min (W) = WOB x f WOB / liter = W / $\dot{V}_E$ WOB total = WOB patient + WOB vent	The energy (pressure gradient) required to take a breath. Normal = 0.6 - 1.0 j (1j = 0.1 kg.m) W / $\dot{V}_E$ closely reflects abnormal pulmonary mechanics.	Intrinsic WOB = energy required to overcome patient's elastic and resistive forces. Extrinsic WOB = energy required to overcome added extrinsic systems
Weaning Equations		
CROP CROP = Cdyn x (PaO_2/PAO_2) x PImax / rate	C = compliance R = rate O = oxygenation P = pressure	< 13 mL/breath/min indicative of weaning failure.
Simplified Weaning Index SWI = f (mech) x (PIP - PEEP / PImax) x ($PaCO_2$ / 40)	Normal = < 9 min	Simplified version of weaning index (WI). Less accurate than WI, but quick and easy. > 11 min indicative of weaning failure
P0.1 / PImax and RSBI (f / V_T): See above		

Equation	Comments	Significance
Perfusion/Hemodynamic Monitoring		
Cardiac Index (CI) CI = CO/BSA	Cardiac output per body size. Normal = 2.5 - 4.4 L/min/m^2 BSA (See Pg 7-28)	More precise measure of pump efficiency than CO. CI 1.8 - 2.5 = moderate cardiac disease CI < 1.8 = severe cardiac disease
Cardiac Output (CO or $\dot{Q}_T$) CO = SV x HR	Normal = 4-8 L/min (at rest) See Fick equation below & Oakes' ***Hemodynamic Monitoring: A Bedside Reference Manual*** for more information.	Amount of blood ejected from heart per minute. Indicator of pump efficiency and a determinant of tissue perfusion.
Coronary Artery Perfusion Pressure (CPP or CAPP) CPP = MAP - PAWP = BPdia - PAWP	Normal = 60-80 mm Hg	Driving pressure of coronary blood flow.
Fick Equation $\dot{V}O_2 = CO \times Ca\text{-}\bar{v}O_2$	See Oakes' ***Hemodynamic Monitoring: A Bedside Reference Manual*** for more info.	Method of measuring cardiac output. Fick estimate: $CO = 125 \times BSA / Ca\text{-}\bar{v}O_2$

Equation	Comments	Significance
Left Ventricular Stroke Work (LVSW) LVSW = ($\overline{BP}$ – PAWP) x SV x 0.0136	Normal = 60-80 gm/m/beat	Measure of pumping function of left ventricle (LV contractility).
Left Ventricular Stroke Work Index (LVSWI) LVSWI = ($\overline{BP}$ – PAWP) x SVI x 0.0136	Normal = 40-75 gm/m/beat/m^2	Measure of pumping function of left ventricle (LV contractility) / body size.
Mean Arterial Blood Pressure ($\overline{BP}$, MAP) $\overline{BP} = 1/3\ PP + BPdia$ $= \frac{BPsys + 2BPdia}{3}$	Normal = 93 mmHg (70-105)	Average driving force of systemic circulation. Determined by cardiac output and total peripheral resistance.
Mean Pulmonary Artery Pressure ($\overline{PAP}$, PAMP) $\overline{PAP}$ = 1/3 pulmPP + PADP	Normal = 10 - 15 mmHg $= \frac{PASP + 2PADP}{3}$	Average driving force of blood from the right heart to left heart.
Pulmonary Vascular Resistance (PVR) $PVR = \frac{PAMP - PAWP}{CO} \times 80$	Normal = 20-250 dynes•sec•cm^{-5} = 0.25-2.5 units (mm Hg/L/min) E.g. $\frac{14\ mm\ Hg - 5\ mm\ Hg}{5\ L/min}$ = 1.8 units	Resistance to RV ejection of blood into pulmonary vasculature. Indicator of RV afterload. mm Hg/L/min x 80 = dynes•sec•cm^{-5}

Equation	Comments	Significance
Pulmonary Vascular Resistance Index (PVRI) $PVRI = \frac{PAMP - PAWP}{CI} \times 80$	Normal = 35-350 dynes•sec•cm^{-5}/m^2	PVR related to body size.
Pulse Pressure (PP) PP = BPsys - BPdia	Normal = 40 mm Hg (20-80)	Difference between BP systolic and BP diastolic.
Rate Pressure Product (RPP) RPP = BPsys x HR	Normal = < 12,000 mm Hg/min	Indirect determinant of $M\dot{V}O_2$.
Right Ventricular Stroke Work (RVSW) = (PAMP - CVP) x SV x 0.0136	Normal = 10-15 gm/m/beat	Measure of pumping function of right ventricle (RV contractility).
Right Ventricular Stroke Work Index (RVSW) = (PAMP - CVP) x SVI x 0.0136	Normal = 4-12 $gm/m/beat/m^2$ = RVSW / BSA	Measure of pumping function of right ventricle (RV contractility) / body size.

Equation	Comments	Significance
Shunt Equation ($\dot{Q}s/\dot{Q}_T$) 1) Classical $\dot{Q}s/\dot{Q}_T = \frac{CcO_2 - CaO_2}{Cc\text{-}\bar{v}O_2}$	Normal = 2-5% CcO_2 = pulmonary capillary blood O_2 content ("ideal") at 100% saturated with alveolar O_2. Cannot be sampled. CcO_2 = (Hgb x 1.34) SaO_2 + (PAO_2 x 0.003)	Indicates ratio of shunted blood (Qs) (blood not participating in gas exchange) to total cardiac output (Q_T). $Qs = Q_T - Qc$ Qs = QSphys = Qsanat + Qscap Indicator or efficiency of pulm system: < 10% = normal lungs 10-20% = minimal effect 20-30% = significant pulm disease > 30% = life-threatening
2) Clinical $\dot{Q}s/\dot{Q}_T = \frac{PA\text{-}aO_2 \times 0.003}{Ca\text{-}\bar{v}O2 + PA\text{-}aO2 \times 0.003}$	Less accurate/easier. Perform breathing ↑ FIO_2 (50% preferred over 100% due to ↑shunting from alveolar collapse) x 20 minutes.	Clinical equation assumes Hgb 100% saturated (PaO_2 > 150). If PaO_2 < 150, then must use classical shunt equation.
3) Estimate $\dot{Q}s/\dot{Q}_T = \frac{PA\text{-}aO2 \times 0.003}{3.5 + PA\text{-}aO2 \times 0.003}$		$Ca\text{-}\bar{v}O_2$ can be assumed if a mixed venous sample cannot be obtained: 4.5 - 5% in patients with good CO and perfusion. 3.5% in critically ill patients.
4) Estimates $\dot{Q}s/\dot{Q}_T = \frac{PA\text{-}aO_2}{20}$ $\dot{Q}s/\dot{Q}_T$ = 5% per every 100 mm Hg below expected	5%/100 mm Hg (2%/50 mm Hg) Most accurate when breathing 100% O_2. Plus normal 2-5%. Estimate good until PaO_2 < 100 mm Hg	Estimate: PaO_2/FIO_2 > 300 = < 15% shunt 200 - 300 = 15 - 20%; < 200 = > 20% shunt

Equation	Comments	Significance
Stroke Volume (SV) SV = CO/HR x 1000	Normal = 60-120 mL/beat	Amount of blood ejected by either ventricle per contraction.
Stroke Volume Index (SVI) SVI = CO/HR x 1000 / BSA	Normal = 35-75 $mL/beat/m^2$	Relates SV to body size.
Systemic Vascular Resistance (SVR) $SVR = \frac{\overline{BP} - CVP}{CO} \times 80$	Normal = 800-1600 $dynes \bullet sec \bullet cm^{-5}$ = 10-20 units (mm Hg/L/min) E.g. $\frac{93\ mm\ Hg - 3\ mm\ Hg}{5\ L/min}$ = 18 units	Resistance to LV ejection of blood into systemic circulation. Indicator of LV afterload. mm Hg/L/min x 80 = $dynes \bullet sec \bullet cm^{-5}$
Systemic Vascular Resistance Index (SVRI) $SVRI = \frac{\overline{BP} - CVP}{CI} \times 80$	Normal = 1400-2600 $dynes \bullet sec \bullet cm^{-5} / m^2$	SVR per body size.
Patient Calculations		
Body Surface Area (BSA) BSA (m^2) = (Ht $(cm)^{0.725}$) x (Wt $(kg)^{0.425}$) x 0.007184	BSA (m^2) = (4 x Kg) + 7 / Kg + 90	Used to determine cardiac index and other hemodynamic parameters. Relates parameters to body size. Kg = 2.2 lbs

Equation	Comments	Significance
Ideal Body Weight (IBW) Hamwi method (see page 10-6 for PBW)	Male: 106 lbs for 5 ft tall. Add 6 lbs/in above 5 ft. 1 Kg = 2.2 lbs	Female: 100 lbs for 5 ft tall. Add 5 lbs/in above 5 ft.
Miscellaneous		
ATPS to BTPS Vol BTPS = Vol ATPS x factor	See Appendix	Correction of lung volumes measured at room temp to body temp.
Fick's Law of Diffusion Diffusion = $\frac{\text{Area x diffusion coefficient x } \Delta P}{\text{Thickness}}$		Gas diffusion rate across the lung membrane.
Gas Laws Dalton's Law: Total P = P1+P2+P3, etc. Boyle's Law: P1 x V1 = P2 x V2 — P and V are inversely related (T constant) Charles' Law: V1/T1 = V2/T2 — V and T are directly related (P constant) Gay-Lussac's Law: P1/T1 = P2/T2 — P and T are directly related (V constant) Combined Gas Law: P1 x V1 / T1 = P2 x V2 / T2		
Graham's Law of Diffusion Coefficient	Diffusion coefficient = $\frac{\text{solubility coefficient}}{\sqrt{\text{gmw}}}$	Rate of gas diffusion is inversely proportional to the square root of its gram molecular weight.

Equation	Comments	Significance
Helium/Oxygen (He/O_2) Flow Conversion	80% He / 20% O_2: actual flow = flow x 1.8 70% He / 30% O_2 = flow x 1.6 60% He / 40% O_2 = flow x 1.4	Conversion is used when an O_2 flow meter is used to measure Heliox flow. Used in patients with obstructive disorders.
Law of LaPlace	P = 2ST / r	P = pressure (dynes/cm^2); r = radius (cm) ST = surface tension (dynes/cm)
Oxygen Blending Ratios FIO_2 desired ↓ 100 ___ air units ___ ___ O2 units ___ 21	Select desired FIO_2. Subtract 100 - FIO_2 = air units Subtract FIO_2 - 20 = O_2 units	To find air/O_2 ratio for desired FIO_2. Air units/O_2 units = air/O_2 ratio E.g: 40% O_2 desired $\frac{100 - 40 = 60}{40 - 20 = 20} = \frac{60}{20} = \frac{3}{1}$

<table>
<tr><th>Equation</th><th>Comments</th><th>Significance</th></tr>
<tr><td>Oxygen Duration Times

Duration of a Cylinder

$\text{Time (min)} = \dfrac{\text{Pcyl} \times \text{CF}}{\text{Flow (L/min)}}$</td><td>$P_{cyl}$ = total pressure in cylinder (psi) – 500 psi (reserve)

CF = conversion factor (L/psi)
$= \dfrac{(\text{ft}^3 \text{ of cyl}) \times 28.3\ \text{L/ft}^3}{\max P_{cyl}}$</td><td>Used to calculate how long a cylinder of O2 gas will last. 500 psi equals reserve.
<table><tr><th>Size</th><th>ft^3</th><th>factor</th></tr><tr><td>A</td><td>2.7</td><td>0.035</td></tr><tr><td>B</td><td>5.3</td><td>0.068</td></tr><tr><td>D</td><td>12.6</td><td>0.16</td></tr><tr><td>E</td><td>22</td><td>0.28</td></tr><tr><td>G</td><td>186</td><td>2.41</td></tr><tr><td>H/K</td><td>244</td><td>3.14</td></tr><tr><td>M</td><td>128</td><td>1.56</td></tr></table></td></tr>
<tr><td>Duration of a Liquid System</td><td>Liquid weight is known:
Duration time (min) =
$\dfrac{344\ \text{L/lb} \times \text{liquid weight (lb)}}{O_2 \text{ flow (L/min)}}$
1 L liquid = 860 L gas
Liquid Wt = Total Wt - Cylinder Wt</td><td>Gauge fraction is known:
Duration time (min) =
$\dfrac{\text{Liquid capacity (L)} \times 860 \times \text{gauge fraction}}{O_2 \text{ flow (L/min)}}$

Note: Does not account for evaporative loss.</td></tr>
</table>

Equation	Comments	Significance
Oxygen Entrainment Ratios $TF = \frac{O_2 \text{ flow} \times 0.79}{FIO_2 - 0.21}$ $FIO_2 = \frac{0.79}{TF / O_2 \text{ Flow}} + 0.21$	TF = total flow in liters (O_2 + air) Mixture = O_2 + air (FIO_2)(Flow) = (1.0)(O_2 Flow) + (0.21)(air Flow)	Determines total flows, entrained flows, or O_2 percent when air and O_2 are entrained together. See O_2 blending ratio above.
Poiseuille's Law $\dot{V} = \frac{\Delta P\ r\ 4\pi}{\mu L 8} = \Delta P\ r^4$	$\dot{V}$ = flow, πP = driving pressure 8 = constant, r = radius of airway π = pi	μ = viscosity of gas L = length of airway
Reynold's Number $Rn = \frac{v \times D \times d}{\mu}$	Rn = Reynold's # v = velocity of fluid D = density of fluid	d = diameter of tube μ = viscosity of fluid Rn < 2000 = laminar flow Rn > 2000 = turbulent
Temperature Conversion	$F = (C^\circ \times 9/5) + 32^\circ$ $C^\circ = (F^\circ - 32) \times 5/9$	See Appendix $K^\circ = C^\circ + 273$

Make It Your Own

Notes Page

Make It Your Own

Notes Page

8 Management

CONTENTS

Emergency Airway Management 8-2
Intubation Procedure 8-2
Successful Intubation Checklist 8-2
End-tidal CO_2 Verification 8-3
Bag and Valve-Mask Ventilation 8-4

Ventilator Management
Ventilation
Improving Ventilation 8-5
Quick Formulas for Calculating 8-5
Permissive Hypercapnia 8-10

Oxygenation
Improving Oxygenation 8-11
Quick Estimates/Formulas for Calculating 8-11
Methods for Improving 8-12
FIO_2 8-12
PEEP/CPAP 8-13
Beneficial/Adverse Effects of PEEP 8-13
Initiating Therapeutic Levels 8-14
Optimal PEEP 8-15
Applied PEEP with auto-PEEP 8-17
Common Parameters in Monitoring 8-18
Weaning PEEP 8-18
Mean Airway Pressure 8-19
Primary Factors Affecting 8-19
Measuring Mean Airway Pressure 8-19
Patient Positioning 8-20
Inverse Ratio Strategies 8-21

Patient-Ventilator Synchrony
Common Signs of Asynchrony 8-22
Typical Causes and Possible Solutions 8-22

Emergency Airway Management

Intubation Procedure

Prepare all equipment, and fully assess the patient prior to intubating:

- Bag and Valve Mask Ventilation (BVM) via O_2 (12+ L/min)
- Laryngoscope handle
- Laryngsocope Blades (Miller or MacIntosh) - check light source
- Endotracheal Tube (several sizes) with stylet
  Use new Endotracheal Tube on each Intubation attempt
- 10 cc Syringe
- Suction equipment
- $ETCO_2$ detector, capnography, EDD, etc. for verifying placement

IMPORTANT CONSIDERATIONS:

- Have all possible equipment at bedside to anticipate difficulties (fiberoptic equipment, bronchoscope, etc.)
- Cautious Rapid Sequence Intubation (RSI) in pts who are obese , pts who are known difficult intubations, etc.
- Pulse Oximetry, Blood Pressure, and EKG must be monitored during intubation. Interrupt attempt if oxygenation/ventilation is needed
- Only direct visualization is completely reliable. Use all possible verification methods. IF IN DOUBT, PULL IT OUT
- Remove tube at once if gurgling in stomach, and no chest expansion

Insertion Depth: Male (21-23 cm); Female (19-21 cm)

Successful Intubation Checklist:

	Lungs: equal + bilateral breath sounds, Chest Expans.
	Abdomen: ↓ sounds in abdom, No ↑ abdom. distention
	Warm air exhaled from ET Tube
	+ $ETCO_2$* (YELLOW is YES, PURPLE is PROBLEM)
	Condensate inside ET Tube
	Improved patient color/SpO_2
	Visualization with Scope
	CXR Verification
	Esophageal Detector Device (EDD) - optional

End-tidal CO_2 Detector ($P_{ET}CO_2$) for Verification

CO_2 Detected	
Tube likely in trachea	May rarely detect CO_2 if tube in esophagus and lg amts of carbonated fluid ingested prior to intubation. This will dissipate after a few ventilations.
CO_2 Not Detected	
Tube is in Esophagus	• Absent Chest Rise • Absent Breath Sounds • Stomach gurgling / distension
Tube is in Trachea ***Verify with multiple other methods***	*Decreased CO_2 IN Lungs:* • Poor blood flow to lungs • Cardiac Arrest • Pulmonary Embolus • IV Bolus of Epinephrine *Decreased CO_2 FROM Lungs:* • Airway Obstruct (Status Asthm., etc.) • Pulmonary Edema • Mucus Plugging
Unclear Where Tube Is	Detector Contaminated with gastric contents or acidic drug
ETCO2 device applied incorrectly, Time	Many disposable devices require "activation" (such as by pulling of paper tab), and may req. a few ventilations to change color

Esophageal Detector Device for Verification

Syringe-Type plunger is attached to ET Tube.	
Able to Pull Back on Plunger	ET Tube likely in trachea (rigid structure of trachea allows for air passage)
Unable to Pull Back on Plunger	ET Tube likely in esophagus (floppy structure of esophagus collapses over end of ET tube)
Caution: May be misleading in morbid obesity, late pregnancy, status asthmaticus, or with copious secretions. Use in Children only if > 20 kg and with perfusing rhythm.	

Bag and Valve Mask Ventilation (BVM)

<table>
<tr><th>Variable</th><th colspan="2">Considerations</th></tr>
<tr><td rowspan="3">Rates</td><td>Most Pts</td><td>10-12 breaths/min (every 5-6 sec) with 1 sec inspiration</td></tr>
<tr><td>COPD
↑ Raw</td><td>6-8 breaths/min (every 7-10 sec) with 1 sec inspir. (avoids auto-PEEP)</td></tr>
<tr><td>CPR</td><td>8-10 breaths/min (permits venous return)</td></tr>
<tr><td rowspan="3">Volumes</td><td colspan="2">Estimated (deliver enough for visible chest rise):</td></tr>
<tr><td>Adult</td><td>500-600 mL (6-7 mL/kg)
1 L Adult Bag: 1/2 - 2/3 vol
2 L Adult Bag: 1/3 vol</td></tr>
<tr><td>Infant/ Child</td><td>Visible Chest Rise
Bag size should be > 450-500 mL</td></tr>
<tr><td>Gas Source</td><td colspan="2">Run >12 L/min of Oxygen (bag inflated). Verify O_2 flowmeter, and hasn't disconnected or is on Air</td></tr>
<tr><td>Personnel</td><td colspan="2">Most effective with 2 Rescuers - 1 opens airway/seals mask, 2nd squeezes bag while both observe chest rise</td></tr>
<tr><td rowspan="6">Cautions</td><td colspan="2">Avoid Hyperinflation</td></tr>
<tr><td colspan="2">Giving > 12 breaths/min (>q 5 sec) may ↑ Intra-thoracic Pressure, ↓ venous return, ↓ CO, and ↓ coronary/cerebral perfusion</td></tr>
<tr><td colspan="2">Gastric inflation</td></tr>
<tr><td colspan="2">Giving large or forceful breaths may cause regur-gitation, aspiration, elevated diaphragm, ↓ lung movement, and ↓ CL</td></tr>
<tr><td colspan="2">Patient Vomits</td></tr>
<tr><td colspan="2">Turn to side, wipe/sx out oral cavity, return to Supine</td></tr>
<tr><td>Inadequate Face/Mask Ventilation</td><td colspan="2">• Absent or ↓: bs, chest movement, expired CO_2
• ↓ SpO_2, Cyanosis
• Excessive gas leak
• Gastric air entry/dilatation
• Hemodyn. changes (↑HR, ↑ BP, arrhythmias)</td></tr>
</table>

Management

Ventilation

Improving Ventilation: $PaCO_2$ (and pH)	
Goal	Maintain adequate CO_2 elimination while protecting the lungs from injury.
Principle	Adequacy of ventilation is mostly determined by minute ventilation, and assessed by $PaCO_2$/pH (Several therapeutic strategies exist, including lung protection) (see Permissive Hypercapnea) $PaCO_2$ and resultant pH are impacted by total ventilation, deadspace, and CO_2 production. They are changed by altering minute ventilaton, deadspace and/or CO_2 production. Note that deadspace is not often used therapeutically anymore.

Quick Formula (Calculating Minute Volume to achieve a $PaCO_2$)
New $\dot{V}_E = \dfrac{\text{Current } \dot{V}_E \times \text{Current } PaCO_2}{\text{Desired } PaCO_2}$

Quick Formula (Calculating Tidal Volume to achieve a $PaCO_2$)*
New $V_T = \dfrac{\text{Current } V_T \times \text{Current } PaCO_2}{\text{Desired } PaCO_2}$

Quick Formula (Calculating RR to achieve a $PaCO_2$)*
New $f = \dfrac{\text{Current } f \times \text{Current } PaCO_2}{\text{Desired } PaCO_2}$

*These formulas assume a patient is on a control-mode of ventilation, not making spontaneous efforts. The formulas can be used only as an estimate in patients with spontaneous breathing patients.

Management

Uncompensated Respiratory Acidosis

↑ $PaCO_2$ with ↓ pH

Increasing Minute Ventilation will blow off more CO_2 (generally)

Mode Type	Strategies
Volume	1. Increase f (be sure to adjust T_I simultaneously to ensure adequate exhalation). See Quick Formula on previous page for calculating f. 2. Increase V_T - use with caution! Most of the time V_T is set by cc/kg IBW, so it is less common to increase V_T.
Pressure	1. Increase f (be sure to adjust T_I simultaneously to ensure adequate exhalation). See Quick Formula on previous page for calculating f. 2. Increase V_T by either increasing Inspiratory Pressure, or increasing T_I. Again, use with caution as V_T is most often set by cc/kg IBW, so it is less common to increase V_T.

Additional Strategies

1) Increase VT_{spont}
   - A) PSV
   - B) Bronchodilation
   - C) Increase ET tube size
   - D) Respiratory muscle conditioning
   - E) Improve nutritional support
2) Decrease mechanical V_D
   - A) Use low compliance circuit
   - B) Cut ET tube shorter
   - C) Tracheostomy
3) High Frequency Ventilation
4) Permissive Hypercapnia (see below)

Uncompensated Respiratory Acidosis

↑ $PaCO_2$ with ↓ pH with adequate/high Minute Ventilation

Increasing Minute Ventilation will blow off more CO_2 (generally)

Potential Causes:

↑ Deadspace (V_D/V_T)	↑ CO_2 production
Possible Causes:	***Possible Causes:***
Air trapping High I:E ratio (e.g., 3:1) Low $\dot{V}_I$ Pulmonary emboli or hypoperfusion Uneven gas distribution (lung pathology)	Burns Fever Hyperthyroidism Multiple surgeries Multiple trauma Sepsis
Possible Solutions:	***Possible Solutions:***
Increase flow Decrease I:E ratio Reposition patient	Correct primary cause Note: Increasing $\dot{V}_E$ further may lead to air trapping and auto-PEEP PSV may be helpful to ↓WOB

Management

Uncompensated Respiratory Alkalosis

↓ $PaCO_2$ and ↑ pH

Note: A Respiratory Alkalosis present in patients "riding the vent" (Total RR = Set RR) is clinician-induced and should be corrected. A Respiratory Alkalosis in a patient who has spontaneous breaths must be further analyzed before fixing - alkalosis in this case is sometimes left uncorrected

Mode Type	Strategies
Volume	1. Decrease *f*. See Quick Formula on previous page for calculating *f*. 2. Decrease V_T - when V_T > Deadspace Ventilation
Pressure	1. Decrease *f*. See Quick Formula on previous page for calculating *f*. 2. Decrease V_T by either decreasing Inspiratory Pressure, or carefully decreasing T_I. Again, use with caution as V_T is most often set by cc/kg IBW, so it is less common to increase V_T.

Additional Strategies

If patient is on A/C, decreasing *f* of mandatory breaths may have no effect. If ↓ V_T and patient increases *f* then :

1) Try PSV or SIMV (allows spontaneous control)
2) Sedate (Use with caution, but consider in patients with extreme agitation, fear, pain, or ↑WOB)
3) Add VD_{mech} (not often used clinically)

If patient is hyperventilating due to hypoxemia, correct the hypoxemia first.

Compensated Metabolic Disorders

The lungs compensate quickly for metabolic disorders, unless beyond their capacity to do so, or when the respiratory system is fully controlled on the ventilator.

Compensated Metabolic Acidosis

↓ $PaCO_2$ and Normal/**↓ pH**
Patient is likely to be hyperventilating on vent

How to Fix: Correct the root cause of the metabolic acidosis when possible. Sodium bicarbonate is sometimes used when clinically significant acidosis, but is used only temporarily until root cause can be addressed.

Compensated Metabolic Alkalosis

↑ $PaCO_2$ and Normal/ ↑ pH
Patient is likely to be hypoventilating on vent

How to Fix: Correct the root cause of the metabolic alkalosis when possible. Few options exist when alkalosis is clinically significant. Caution should be used with increasing minute ventilation (CO_2 will be high) as this will worsen alkalosis, which may result in cardiac dysrhythmias, seizures, etc.

Permissive Hypercapnia	
Definition	Therapeutically allowing the CO_2 to increase (and thus pH to drop to acidosis) by limiting ventilatory support - usually V_T
Goal	Lung protection (prevent damage to alveoli)
Indications	Many clinicians employ permissive hypercapnia in the majority of critical care patients (prophphylactic) Any time Pplat is rising (close to 30 cmH_2O)
Contraindications (Relative)	Cerebral traumas, hemorrhage, CNS lesions (↑CO_2 → cerebral vasodilation → ↑ ICP) and CV instability (↑ $PaCO_2$ and ↓ pH may lead to ↓ myocardial contractility, arrhythmias, and/or vasodilation)
How To	Ventilate with low V_T (4-7 cc/kg IBW) to keep Pplat < 30 cmH_2O. 4 cc is lower end of V_T range due to anatomic deadspace of around 2 cc/kg IBW $PaCO_2$ is allowed to ↑ to 50 - 100 mmHg and pH is allowed to ↓ to 7.15 - 7.20. Introduction of hypercapnia should be gradual (< 10 mmHg/hr)
Considerations	Patients may require increased sedation to tolerate lower V_T strategy PEEP should be optimized to maintain lung recruitment with lower V_T. Consider Sodium Bicarbonate or other intervention for patients with pH < 7.15
Physiologic Effects	CNS depression, May ↑ ICP. May reduce PaO_2, Right shift of Oxyhemoglobin Curve, Dyspnea (stimulation of ventilation), pulmonary vasoconstriction, CV effects (hypotension)

Oxygenation

Improving Oxygenation: PaO_2 (SaO_2, SpO_2)	
Goal	To maintain adequate O_2 delivery to the tissues while ventilating with the lowest possible F_IO_2 and pressures.
Principle	PaO_2 is affected primarily by F_IO_2, $\overline{P}aw$ (V_T, PIP, PEEP, T_I, $\dot{V}I$, $\dot{V}I$ waveform) and cardiovascular disease (i.e., optimizing lung volume and V/Q matching). Adequate O_2 delivery to tissues is dependent on F_IO_2, CO, and CaO_2.

Quick Estimates of Oxygenation Status:

P/F ratio = PaO_2 / F_IO_2

- PaO_2 is the amount of oxygen in the arteries
- FIO_2 is the amount of oxygen in the alveoli (roughly, of course)
- The ratio estimates how well oxygen is getting from alveoli to the arteries.
- Normal is approximately 500

Oxygen Index (OI) = $\frac{F_IO_2 \times \bar{P}aw \times 100}{PaO_2}$ F_IO_2 is a decimal!

OI again estimates the amount of oxygen that goes from alveoli to blood, but takes into account mean airway pressure, which we know is greatly impacted by factors like PEEP. Thus, the OI can be considered a more powerful estimate of oxygenation.

Quick Formula (Calculating New F_IO_2 to alter PaO_2)
New F_IO_2 = $\frac{\text{Desired } PaO_2 \times \text{Known } F_IO_2}{\text{Known } PaO_2}$

Management

Methods for Improving Oxygenation

1. Increase FIO_2 (↑ O_2 tension/gradient)
2. Optimize PEEP (eliminate auto-PEEP, ↑ FRC, ↓ shunting)
3. Optimize Mean Airway Pressure (Paw) (↑ FRC)
4. Position Patient (optimize V/Q matching)
5. Inverse Ratio Ventilation (↑ FRC)

1. F_IO_2	
Goal	Use the minimum amount of supplemental oxygen necessary to maintain adequate oxygenation (not necessarily normal oxygenation)
Principle	This is a major determinant of oxygenation, increasing the $P(A\text{-}a)O_2$ gradient, which usually results in a greater PaO_2.
Clinical Notes	Increase F_IO_2 incrementally. High F_IO_2 over time may lead to Oxygen Toxicity, so the overall goal is to maintain < 0.50 when possible, with conservative PaO_2 goals around 60-80 torr.

2. PEEP	
Goal	OPTIMAL PEEP which: ↑ **PaO_2** – ↓ shunt effect, ↑ FRC, and ↑ C, allowing for the reduction of F_IO_2 and its complications. ↓ **WOB** – Unload the inspiratory muscles (esp. in acute exacerbation of COPD).
Principle	Determinant of oxygenation by affecting Paw.
Clinical Notes	Maintains pressures above ambient pressure during the expiratory phase to prevent collapse of smaller airways and unstable alveoli.
Contrain-dications	**Absolute**: Tension Pneumothorax Untreated Pneumothorax (significant in size) **Relative**: • Barotrauma • Bronchopulmonary fistula • Pre-existing hyper-inflation (COPD, etc.) • Hypovolemia • Recent lung surgery • Unilateral lung disorders

Beneficial Effects of Appropriate PEEP

↑ $\overline{P}aw$ ↑ C_L ↑ PaO_2 (for a given F_IO_2) ↓ WOB

↑ V/Q (the stabilization of collapsing alveoli resulting in improved gas distribution and ↓ R-L shunting).

↑ FRC (which may include recruitment of collapsed alveoli)

↓ Lung injury (minimizes shear forces)

PEEP may be beneficial in patients with CHF by ↓ preload and afterload.

Potential Adverse Effects of PEEP

Alveolar over-distension (volutrauma – which is proportional to lung disease, over-distension, and pressure), ↑ WOB, ↑ V_D/V_T.

CV Effects are dependent on PEEP level, C_{LT}, and CV status. The greatest effect (↓ venous return and CO) is when C_L is high, Ccw is low, and CV reserve is low.

Renal function - May ↓ renal and portal blood flow, hence ↓ UO.

ICP - When PEEP decreases venous return, ICP may ↑. Usually clinically insignificant unless ICP is already elevated. Head elevation may offset PEEP effect.

Management

Initiate PEEP/CPAP Therapy

1. Increase PEEP incrementally if not performing Optimal PEEP maneuver (see below) - usually by 3-5 cmH2O every 10-15 minutes
2. Monitor patient closely after each change, including vital signs (especially BP); ventilator parameters, and appearance.
3. Assess after a period of time - as appropriate - ABGs, Oxygenation, Ventilation, Hemodynamic Parameters.

PEEP Ranges

Level	Purpose
Low PEEP: 3 - 5 cmH_2O	Physiologic – to preserve patient's normal FRC
Moderate PEEP: 5 - 15 cmH_2O	Treat refractory hypoxemia caused by ↑ intra-pulmonary shunting with ↓ FRC and ↓ C. Most common range used for acute lung injury.
High PEEP: > 15 cmH_2O	Often reserved for severe lung injury
Optimal PEEP	See below

Definition: Best PEEP, preferred PEEP, therapeutic PEEP – the level of PEEP at which O_2 delivery to the tissues is maximized. Optimal PEEP generally correlates with the point where alveolar de-recruitment does not occur. That is:

The lowest PEEP level at which maximum beneficial effects occur:	With the least cardio-pulmonary side effects:
↑ O_2 transport (↑ PaO_2, $P\bar{v}O_2$, O_2 Sat) ↑FRC, ↓ Shunt ↑ Compliance	↓ venous return ↓ CO, ↓ BP ↑Shunt, ↑V_D/V_T Barotrauma

Management

Optimal PEEP Determination

1. Use of Pressure-Volume (P-V) Loop

Goal: Set PEEP between the Lower Inflection Point and Upper Inflection Point (see diagram on next page)

Procedure:

- Consider administration of a dose of paralytic (with sedation) in order to obtain accurate P-V loop.
- Identify Lower and Upper Inflection Points (LIP and UIP) on loop.
- Choose a PEEP that is approximately 2 cmH_2O above the LIP, always ensuring it is below the UIP.

2. Incremental PEEP study

This bedside procedure is perhaps the most simple.

Procedure:

- Increase PEEP by about 3 cmH_2O at a time, calculating static compliance (inspiratory hold) at each step.
  $C_{stat} = V_T/(P_{plat} - PEEP)$
- Use the level of applied PEEP that resulted in the best compliance (largest C_{stat}).

Alternative: Increase PEEP by 2-3 cmH_2O at a time, carefully observing SpO_2, V_T, and BP. Optimal PEEP is determined to be the minimum PEEP which increases V_T and potentially SpO_2 without causing a decrease in BP (suggesting you are over-distending).

3. Oxygenation PEEP Study

After a goal PaO_2 is determined, PEEP is titrated to achieve the PaO_2 with an $F_IO_2 < 0.50$.

4. Esophageal Pressure

Using an esophageal balloon catheter, this estimates pleural pressure:

Transpulmonary P = Paw - Ppleural

Goal = End-Inspiratory Transpulmonary Pressure < 25 cmH_2O

No specific PEEP maneuver is preferred over another in current literature. Regardless of method used, the clinician should work to ensure safety of the lungs, and carefully monitor parameters.

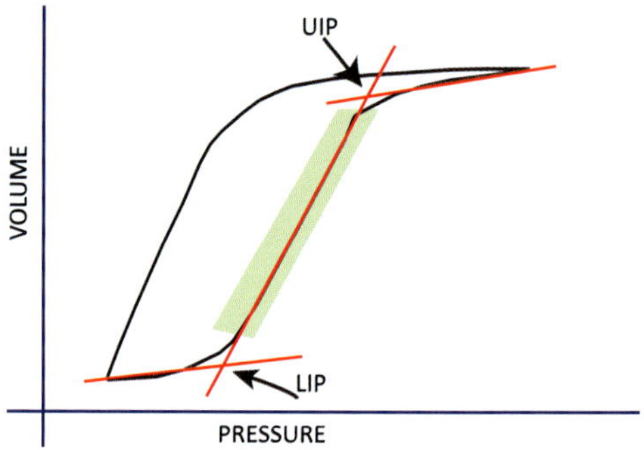

Understanding the P-V Loop and PEEP:

1. The steep part of the curve represents rapid increases in Volume with small pressure changes, implying best compliance as the lungs accept volume easily.
2. The flattened sections represent areas where it takes greater pressures to move small volumes of air (the cost of ventilation, and the risk of lung damage, is high):

   Lower: Lower flattened section suggests areas of the lungs that are closing and opening, which results in atelectrauma. These are separated in the above diagram by the Lower Inflection Point (LIP).

   Upper: Upper flattened section ("duckbill"), when present, suggests over-distension, which can lead to barotrauma (damage caused by excessive pressure). PEEP should always be set below the Upper Inflection Point (UIP).
3. The slope of the curve provides information about lung compliance. Less steep curves suggest poor compliance (it always takes a fair amount of pressure to deliver a volume)
4. Ideally this curve is captured with no patient contribution, meaning it is most accurate when a patient is given a single-dose of a paralytic. Note that the LIP in particular is not always discernible.

Using Applied PEEP in the presence of Auto–PEEP

Applied PEEP (extrinsic PEEP) may be applied up to 80% of measured auto-PEEP. This technique is recommended for patients with auto-PEEP who are having trouble triggering the ventilator.

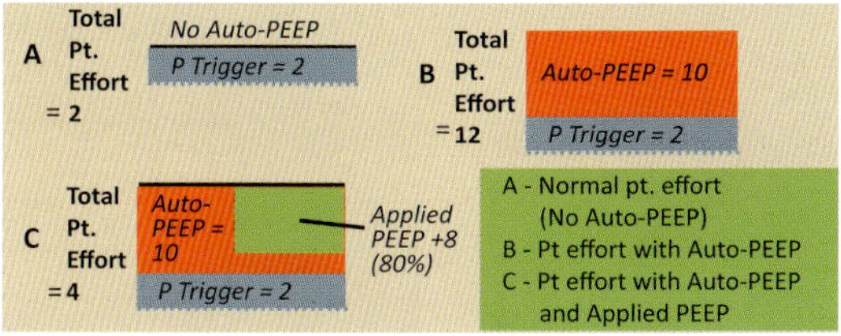

Theory: up to 80% of applied PEEP only affects the circuit and airway pressures and not alveolar pressures. It works to equilibrate trapped pressure and circuit pressure.

Note: Applied PEEP > 80% will begin to ↑ Palv with CV effects.

Two Techniques

1) Esophageal balloon
2) Incremental Approach

   ↑ Applied PEEP in increments of 2 - 5 cmH_2O until every patient-triggering-effort initiates a ventilator breath.

Signs of Excessive Applied PEEP

↑ dyspnea, ↓ BP, worsening signs of hyperinflation

- See Oakes' ***Hemodynamic Monitoring: A Bedside Reference Manual***, for a thorough reference to hemodynamic changes with PEEP and zone changes.
- **PEEP /F_IO_2 Algorithm** – *For the Algorithm used in the NIH ARDS Network MV Protocol see ARDS, Chapter 10.*
- *See page 11-3:* **Details of Auto-PEEP, including identifying, measuring, and reducing Auto-PEEP**

Common Parameters for Measuring and Monitoring PEEP

Ventilation and Oxygenation

Ventilation		Oxygenation	
Parameter	**Desired Goal**	**Parameter**	**Desired Goal**
Breath sounds	Appropriate	PaO_2	60-100 mmHg on $F_IO_2 \le 0.4$
V_T, *f*, $\dot{V}_E$	Appropriate	SaO_2	90-97% @ normal pH
PIP, P_{plat}, PEEP	Minimal	F_IO_2	Decreasing
Cdyn	Improving	PaO_2/F_IO_2	> 300 mmHg
Cstat	Improving	$P(A\text{-}a)O_2$	Decreasing
Raw	Decreasing	PaO_2/PAO_2	Increasing
$PaCO_2$, pH	Appropriate	Shunt (Q_S/Q_T)	< 15%
$P(a\text{-}et)CO_2$	Decreasing		

Hemodynamics

O_2 Transport	≈ 1000 mL/min (5L x 20 vol%)
CO	Increasing or < 20% decrease
BP	Adequate or < 20% decrease
PA Pressures	Appropriate
PAOP	No change (marked ↑ may indicate over-inflation of alveoli; marked ↓ may indicate ↓ blood flow due to ↓ CO)
$P\bar{v}O_2$	Increasing and > 28 mmHg
$S\bar{v}O_2$	Increasing and > 50%
$C(a\text{-}\bar{v})O_2$	Decreasing

Weaning PEEP

- Top priorities: ↓ plat to < 30 cmH_2O, ↓ PEEP to < 15 cmH_2O, ↓ F_IO_2 to < 0.5
- Do not abruptly withdraw PEEP (except hemodynamic compromise)
- ↓ PEEP in increments (usually 2 cmH_2O) every 1-6 hours
- If PaO_2 ↓ > 20% after PEEP wean, return PEEP to previous level

3. Mean Airway Pressure ($\overline{P}aw$ or MAWP or MAP or mPAW)	
Goal	Achieve adequate oxygenation with the lowest possible pressures and F_IO_2 without impairing CV function or injurying the lungs
Principle	Paw is an important determinant of oxygenation $PaO_2 \sim \overline{P}aw$ (until overdistension occurs - see pg 8-17)
Indication	↑ Paw is indicated for patients with ↓ lung volumes and refractory hypoxemia (does not respond to increasing the F_IO_2) Refractory Hypoxemia = $PaO_2 < 60$ mmHg on $F_IO_2 > 0.6$

Primary Factors Affecting $\overline{P}aw$ (in probable order of influence)

- PEEP
- PIP
- T_I
- f (↓ T_E)
- $\dot{V}_I$
- $\dot{V}_I$ waveform

Clinical Note: Limit T_I to the maximum that does not cause auto-PEEP.
If auto-PEEP present: In VV: auto-PEEP → ↑ Palv (V_T constant)
In PV: auto-PEEP → ↓ V_T (Palv constant)

Potential Risks of ↑ $\overline{P}aw$ = barotrauma, ↓ CO

Measurement Of $\overline{P}aw$

Automatically calculated by ventilator	Manually calculated
Note: this value usually doesn't include any auto-PEEP	$\overline{P}aw = (PIP - PEEP) \times (T_I / T_{total}) + PEEP$ (figuring a constant flow, VV breath and PEEP includes auto-PEEP)

Management

4. Patient Positioning	
Goal	Improve V/Q and FRC by placing patient in various positions - usually either lateral (right side down or left side down) or by proning patient (stomach down)
Principle	This may assist with oxygenation by aligning perfusion (blood will go wherever gravity takes it - down) WITH ventilation (placing the better lung regions where the best perfusion is). You are aligning good lung with good perfusion, as much as possible. BLU GLD (Blue Gold) = Bad Lung UP, Good Lung DOWN (Except with pulm hemorrhage, lung abscess)
Contrain-dication	**Absolute**: Spinal cord instability **Relative**: Thoracic/Abdominal surgeries (recent) Hemodynamic/Cardiovascular instability
Clinical Notes	• Careful monitoring of ventilator parameters and patient deterioration, complications, line/tube placement, etc., is essential during and directly following repositioning • Improvement is most likely within 30 minutes

Procedure:

- Ensure team members are in place (including 1 person in charge of monitoring secure airway/vent circuit)
- Unhook all leads/lines as necessary
- Gently place pt. on side
- Verify status of pt./equipment/lines
- Place pt. in prone position
- Turn patient's head towards the ventilator
- Reattach and verify all leads/lines - including assuring that the ET tube/head are not compressed
- Do a complete ventilator-patient check, including breath sounds
- Again verify vital signs and hemodynamic status

5. Inverse Ratio Ventilation (IRV) **Not Typically Used (as a mode) in Current Clinical Practice**	
Goal	Setting I:E ratio with T_I being greater than T_E (I:E ratio > 1:1)
Principle	Increasing T_I to ↑ $\overline{P}aw$ and recruit and keep alveoli open for extended periods in order to improve V/Q, without overinflating normal alveolar units.
Indication	When conventional ventilator strategies with optimal PEEP have resulted in P_{plat} > 30 cmH_2O, without providing acceptable PaO_2/F_IO_2 values. Primary use is in patients with ARDS.
Risks	• Auto-PEEP (dynamic hyperinflation) • ↑ PIP in Volume-IRV • ↓ V_T in Pressure-IRV • ↓ $\dot{V}_E$ (↓ V_T or air-trapping) • ↑ PIP • ↓ Cardiac Output
Strategy	↑ T_I in 0.1 – 0.2 sec increments until either PaO_2/F_IO_2 goal is achieved or air-trapping develops. When I:E ratio exceeds 1:1, patients may require sedation and paralysis. **T_I May be Lengthened by:** ↑ Set T_I ↓ $\dot{V}_I$ (VV) Decelerating $\dot{V}_I$ pattern (VV) Inspiratory Pause
Clinical Notes	• Some specialty modes (APRV, BiVent, BiLevel) are basically IRV, but allow for spontaneous breaths during the extended T_I, which may improve synchrony. • Studies have not demonstrated any advantage of using IRV over other methods, but risks are greater (Auto-PEEP, ↑ PIP, ↓ CO, ↓ synchrony)

Patient-Ventilator Synchrony

Often referred to as "fighting the vent", dyssynchrony or asycnhrony. This refers to any time the ventilator fails to deliver what the patient desires.

Common Signs of Asynchrony

Signs include any distress, but include:

- ↑ WOB (mild-severe)
- Paradoxical Breathing (more severe)
- ↑ RR, ↑ HR, ↑ BP
- Graphic Abnormalities (double-stacking, etc.)

*The best way to detect presence and cause of dysynchony is for the clinician to spend time at the bedside carefully analyzing graphics, and watching the patient and ventilator simultaneously. Sometimes the best way to optimize synchrony is to use *trial-and-error* by making small changes and watching for response.

Typical Factors Affecting Patient-Ventilator Interaction

Strategies for discovering and addressing each are on the following pages

- Artificial Airway
- Auto-PEEP (including I:E ratio)
- Exhalation Valve
- Humidity/Humidifiers
- Trigger Sensitivity
- Mode of Ventilation (Mode Dysynchrony)
- Improper Flow (Flow Dysynchrony)
- Improper Cycle (Cycle Dysynchrony)

Artificial Airway

Increases resistance and work of breathing

Common Causes	Potential solutions
ET Tube size too small	• Start with a fairly large ET Tube size (consider 7.5 for women, 8.0 for men) • Consider tube exchange if ↑ WOB and pt has unusually small airway placed • Consider tube compensation (a variable form of Pressure Support), if available
Patient biting on tube (insert suction catheter to verify patency)	• Consider bite block • Carefully consider sedation level
Secretions in Airway (look at graphics, auscultate)	• Suction as needed • Consider bronchoscopy if particularly copious • Consider Heated Humidity if on an HME and thick secretions

Management

Auto-PEEP (Air trapping)

Increases WOB and asynchrony by flattening the diaphragm, affecting respiratory muscle function, and requiring greater effort to trigger the ventilator.

Common Causes	Potential solutions
Underlying Disease Process (COPD, Asthma, etc.)	• See individual diseases for strategies • Verify expiratory flow returns to baseline (using graphics) • Extend I:E ratio to 1:4 or 1:5
Improperly set I:E ratio	Verify that I:E ratio is adequate, reset TI if necessary

Expiratory (Demand) Valves

Pressure-triggered mechanical demand valves often require large pressure drops to open the valves.

Common Causes	Potential solutions
Valve failing to open appropriately	Use flow-triggered system or Add 5 cmH2O to a demand-flow system
Valve sticking due to aerosolized drugs	For drugs known to cause sticking consider changing expiratory filter regularly, or even using two filters

Humidifiers

Increases resistance and work of breathing

Common Causes	Potential solutions
Bubble-through humidifiers with proximal sensitivity can increase resistance and WOB	Use passover or wick-type humidifiers
HME in patients with secretions that continually collect in HME (increases WOB)	Consider Heated Humidifier
Excessive condensate (rain-out) in Heated Humidity	• Verify correct placement/fit of temperature probes • Verify ambient conditions are optimal (no fan blowing on circuit, etc.) • Ensure circuit positioned to minimize collection of condensate

Trigger Sensitivity

May lead to either auto-triggering (too sensitive) or locking patient out (double-stacking, ↑ WOB)

Common Causes	Potential solutions
Leak (Auto-Triggering)	• Verify no leak systematically (disconnect patient from circuit if necessary) • With Noninvasive, verify appropriate mask size and fit for patient
Improper trigger sensitivity or type	• Consider flow trigger when available - this is generally easier to trigger than pressure • Use the most sensitive setting possible without causing auto-triggering • Watch patient's abdomen - as soon as effort is made by patient the ventilator should trigger. If not patient is being "locked out".
Auto-PEEP	If changing to flow does not help or is not possible, consider matching up to 80% of auto-PEEP with Ventilator PEEP
Flow Sensor Malfunction	• Some ventilators use flow sensors, which can quickly become affected by secretions/condensate/placement. • Verify flow sensor is operational, calibrate if able to, consider replacing
Cardiogenic Oscillations	If too sensitive, particularly with bounding heart rate, the ventilator may auto-trigger. Consider changing to a pressure trigger.
Miscellaneous	Inline nebulizers, CPT, etc. (switch to Pressure Trigger during Tx)

Mode Dysynchrony (Ventilatory Support)

Mode dysynchrony occurs when the ventilator is providing too little or too much support for the patient

Common Causes	Potential solutions
Too much support While higher control modes may rest respiratory muscles, it may also lead to atrophy, and may be uncomfortable for patients with any spontaneous drive	• Avoid using purely control modes of ventilation which "lock" the patient out • Use modes that provide adequate support while allowing for spontaneous triggering • Assess regularly for appropriateness to wean
Inadequate support Leads to fatigue	Differentiate between patient inability and other factors like anxiety which may also cause dyssynchrony
Unpredictable Support May lead to dysynchrony - can be thought of as "neural dyssynchrony" as the brain isn't sure whether the next breath will be ventilator-driven or spontaneous	This particularly occurs with SIMV. Consider using Pressure Support Ventilation with adequate Pressure Support level (titrate to reasonable RR and V_T)

Management

Flow Dysynchrony ($\dot{V}_I$ *in VV*)

Inadequate flow leads to an increased WOB

Common Causes	Potential solutions
High demand patients may require 60-100 L/min.	• Assess adequacy of machine flow by observing airway pressure waveform (see Chapter 6). • Adjust $\dot{V}_I$ until airway pressure waveform is restored to normal. • In PV, too long of an inspiratory rise time may lead to ↑ WOB.

Cycle Dysynchrony (TI or Cycle)

Inspiratory Time is set inappropriately usually - patient wants a longer breath, or a shorter breath

Common Causes	Potential solutions
Most commonly, the patient attempts to exhale prior to the termination of machine inspiration. In PV: T_I is set too long In VV: The flow cycle is prolonged	Assess and ensure T_I (set or $\dot{V}_I$ result) is adequate to meet patient's demand.

Make It Your Own

Notes Page

9 Non-Invasive Ventilation

CONTENTS

Acute Management

Management Algorithm *(Acute)* 9-2
Contraindications 9-3
Improvement Criteria 9-3
Indications by Disease 9-4
Treatment Failure Factors (Issues) 9-7
Complications 9-8

Chronic Management

Indications by Disease 9-9
Contraindications 9-9

General Considerations

Management of Patient and NPPV 9-10
Monitoring for Success 9-11
Choosing the Delivery System 9-12
Choosing the Interface 9-13

Other terms and abbreviations used:

Bilevel positive airway pressure
BiPAP (Brand name: Respironics)
Non-invasive ventilation (NIV)
Non-invasive positive pressure ventilation (NIPPV, NPPV)

Definitions:

NPPV: Any form of ventilatory support applied without the use of an endotracheal/tracheal tube: it provides two levels of pressure (I and E) to the airway, which are triggered by the patient or by the ventilator (time) depending on the mode utilized.

Noninvasive Continuous Positive Airway Pressure (CPAP): Technically not a form of noninvasive positive pressure ventilation. It is the application of continuous positive airway pressure throughout the ventilatory cycle.

Inspiratory Positive Airway Pressure (IPAP): The higher pressure level of the two pressures of NPPV.

Expiratory Positive Airway Pressure (EPAP): The lower pressure level of the two pressures of NPPV.

NPPV Management

(Acute Respiratory Failure)

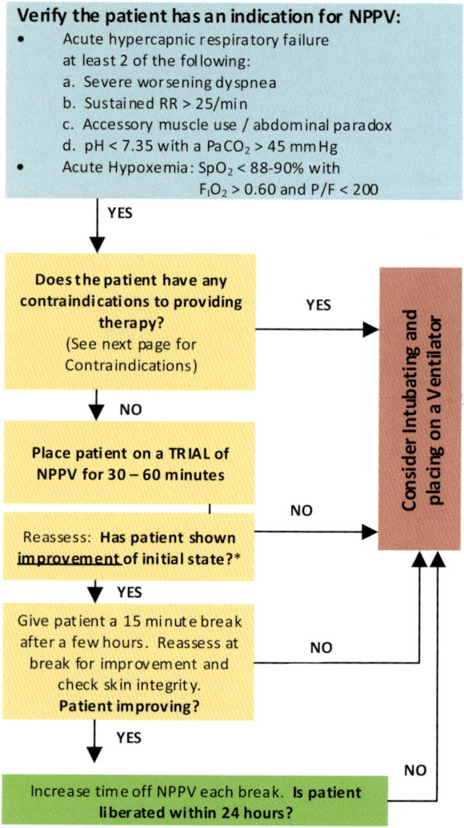

* See next page for general improvement criteria

Contraindications to Providing NPPV

Absolute

1. Apnea
2. Cardiopulmonary arrest
3. Facial burns
4. Facial or cranial trauma
5. Fixed upper airway obstruction
6. Hemodynamic instability/arrhythmias
7. Inability to protect airway/vomiting (risk of aspiration)
8. Need for immediate intubation and airway protection
9. Severe epistaxis
10. Severe respiratory acidosis (pH < 7.20)
11. Upper gastrointestinal (GI) bleeding

Relative

1. Anxiety
2. Bowel obstruction
3. Claustrophobia
4. Copious secretions
5. Inability to clear secretions
6. Inability to cooperate or tolerate interface
7. Severe illness (high APACHE score)

NPPV General Improvement Criteria:

Improvement should be obvious within a relatively short period. Failure to improve (e.g., the patient's clinical state is unchanged) should also be considered as failure, and the patient considered for invasive ventilation.

- Patient: ↓ RR, ↓ WOB, ↓ dyspnea, synchronization with NPPV.
- Improvement in $PaCO_2$ and pH
- Improvement in P/F ratio secondary to lung recruitment

Indications by Disease

Diagnosis	Level of evidence to support use A = Multiple controlled trials B = A single supportive controlled trial C = Uncontrolled trials and case reports	Comments
Acute Exacerbation of COPD	A	• NPPV should be a primary intervention • Most studies showed a reduction in intubations, mortality rates and length of stay • Used for acute exacerbations; not mild cases • Increased success when patient's pH < 7.30 • IPAP assists inhalation/EPAP used to counterbalance "auto-PEEP" • May be used to "buy time" while other therapies take effect
Cardiogenic Pulmonary Edema	A	• Evidence for NPPV and CPAP equal • May be used to "buy time" while other therapies take effect • If hypercapnic, and using CPAP, switch to NPPV
Facilitation of Weaning (COPD patients)	A	• Only used in pts who would otherwise be candidates for NPPV • Used in patients who fail multiple spontaneous breathing trials • Used as a bridge to total liberation
Immuno-compromised Patients	A	• NPPV should be considered early in respiratory failure episode. • These patients have poor outcomes when invasively ventilated. • NPPV offers an option to prevent potentially fatal complications of NPPV (e.g. nosocomial pneumonia)

Diagnosis	Level of evidence to support use A = Multiple controlled trials B = A single supportive controlled trial C = Uncontrolled trials and case reports	Comments
Asthma Exacerbations	B	• NPPV may improve gas exchange and avoid intubations • Can be used initially to reverse airway obstruction more rapidly • NPPV may increase aerosol medication delivery
Extubation Failure	B	• May be used to avoid reintubation • Patients should be monitored closely and intubated when needed if NPPV attempt has failed
Pneumonia	B	• Patients with acute exacerbation of COPD • If progresses to ALI/ARDS, intubate after 1 hour, if patient not improving
Postoperative Respiratory Failure	B	• Prevent postoperative complications after high-risk surgeries • Treat postoperative respiratory failure • Prophylactically treat obese patients following bariatric surgery • Improve oxygenation in CABG patients
ALI/ARDS	C	• Monitor patients closely • Intubate after 1 hour if patient not improving
Cystic Fibrosis	C	• Used as a bridge to transplantation in patients who deteriorate • Treat acute on chronic hypercapnic respiratory failure

Diagnosis	Level of evidence to support use A = Multiple controlled trials B = A single supportive controlled trial C = Uncontrolled trials and case reports	Comments
Do-not-intubate Patients	C	• Very controversial subject • Cause of acute respiratory failure should be reversible such as CHF or COPD. • Used to bridge through the acute illness • Patients have a better prognosis if patient is awake and has a cough. • Patients, family and caregivers should specifically discuss and understand therapy goals and discontinue therapy if goals are not being achieved. • Goal Categories: *(SCCM 2007)* 1. NPPV without preset limits on the provision of advanced life support 2. NPPV for patients who decline ET intubation and invasive MV 3. NPPV as a comfort measure for patients who decline ET intubation
Trauma	C	• May be used in some patients with chest wall injuries. • Not to be used in respiratory-related burn patients
Upper Airway Obstruction	C	• Contraindicated for patients with tight, fixed upper airway obstruction • May be attempted for reversible upper airway obstruction such as post-extubation glottic edema in conjunction with Heliox and/or aerosolized medications.

Overall Issues with NPPV for Treatment of Acute Respiratory Failure

Goals of NPPV in Acute Respiratory Failure	• Avoid intubation and its complications • Improve or stabilize gas exchange • Optimize patient comfort • Reduce work of breathing • Relieve dyspnea
Clinical benefits of NPPV in Acute Respiratory Failure	• Decreases need for sedation • Improves patient comfort • Preserves airway defenses/speech/swallowing • Reduces incidence of nosocomial pneumonia • Reduces mortality • Reduces the need for intubation • Shortens Length of Stay (LOS)
Factors Associated with Predicting Successful NPPV Therapy	• Ability to control secretions • Air leak well controlled • Appropriate level of consciousness • Hypercapnic RF (vs. Hypoxemic RF) • Improvement in pH, $PaCO_2$, respiratory rate, and accessory muscle use after 1 hour of NPPV
Factors Associated with NPPV Treatment Failure	• Deterioration in patient's condition • Deteriorating level of consciousness • Development of complications • Development of new symptoms • Failure to alleviate symptoms • Failure to improve/deterioration in ABGs • Patient refusal • Poor patient tolerance

Complications of NPPV	*Minor:* Air leaks that affect ventilation/pt. comfort Dry upper airway Eye irritation secondary to air leaks (conjunctivitis) Gastric distention General discomfort Patient ventilatory asynchrony Sinus congestion Skin reddening and breakdown ***Major:*** (infrequent) Aspiration (especially with full face masks) Hypotension Pneumothorax

NPPV Management
(Chronic Respiratory Failure)

Chronic conditions where ventilatory support could offer benefit (ventilatory muscle rest, lowering $PaCO_2$), but where cessation of NPPV does not cause an immediate life-threatening risk.

Indications by Disease Category

Disease	Comments
Restrictive Thoracic Disease Chronic hypoventilation syndromes secondary to: • Chest wall or spinal deformity • Idiopathic hypoventilation • Neuromuscular disease • Obesity	May respond gradually over weeks after initiating nocturnal NPPV A mouth piece interface may be tolerated by patients with severe neuromuscular disease who have very low or no Vital Capacity ALS patients with hypercapnia and orthopnea have good prediction of success using NPPV
Chronic Obstructive Pulmonary Disease (COPD)	Very controversial as far as routine use in non-acute exacerbation of COPD
Obstructive Sleep Apnea	Used for patients who cannot tolerate nasal CPAP alone.

Contraindications to Using NPPV Chronically

- Unable to protect airway due to swallowing issues or excessive secretions and a poor cough
- Unable to properly fit interface
- Rapidly progressive neuromuscular disease with bulbar dysfunction
- Unmotivated/uncooperative patient

Management of Patient and NPPV

Therapy Phase	Management
Initiating	• Clinician must take ample time to spend with the patient for optimal success • Explain therapy to patient • Begin at low settings (EPAP 4-5 cmH_2O, IPAP 6-10 cmH_2O) • Place mask gently on patient's face, perhaps allow patient to hold mask on his own face • Do not strap mask on until patient comfortable with pressure • Increase settings as needed and as patient tolerates • Heated humidity is recommended for all patients on NPPV, but is absolutely clinically indicated within several hours following initiation
Managing	• To increase ventilation (*to change pressure support level): Increase IPAP or Decrease EPAP • To decrease ventilation (*to change pressure support level): Decrease IPAP or Increase EPAP • To improve trigger dysynchrony: *Attempt to increase EPAP (If the same PS is desired, clinician must increase IPAP the same increments as the EPAP) *If using a critical care ventilator simply change PS level to affect ventilation and change PEEP to address trigger asynchrony
Weaning	• Begin by decreasing F_IO_2 and pressure as tolerated • Remove NPPV from patient for short breaks and monitor for the need to restart therapy • Breaks may be lengthened to wean further

Monitoring for Success (Type-1)

- Once NPPV is initiated, close observation is required to assess efficacy.
- Rapid improvement should occur (1-2 hours) by the following signs:
- *Patient comfort:* ↓ RR, ↓ use of accessory muscles, ↓ dyspnea, synchronization with NPPV.
- *Improvement in $PaCO_2$ / respiratory acidosis*

Criteria for stopping NPPV attempts and initiating alternative therapy (ET intubation):

- barotrauma
- failure of indications to improve
- hemodynamic instability
- hypercapnia
- inability to accept any of the interfaces attempted
- inability to clear secretions
- pulmonary emboli
- sepsis
- worsening agitation
- worsening mental status
- worsening oxygenation.

Clinical effectiveness is assessed by:

- Improved oximetry
- Improved clinical assessment
- An elevated $PaCO_2$ does not have to drop, however progressive hypercapnia with the application of NPPV indicates failure.

Choosing a Ventilator for Use in NPPV

Type of Ventilator*	Advantages	Disadvantages
Critical Care Ventilators	Any critical care ventilator can be adapted for NPPV use Multiple modes available (pressure support used majority of the time) 21-100% FIO_2 via blender Minimizes CO_2 rebreathing due to dual limb circuit Accurate tracking of V_T and $\dot{V}_E$	Confusion concerning masks and settings if clinicians are used to only using portable bilevel ventilators Limits availability of critical care ventilator Some ventilators may not be as sensitive as portable devices are for leak compensation
Portable Bilevel Ventilators	Most are excellent at leak compensation Portable and ease of use for chronic care	Unable to deliver accurate or high F_IO_2 (not including Respironic's BiPAP Vision/V60) Only one or two modes of ventilation available not including CPAP May rebreath CO_2 due to single limb circuit

* See ventilator manufacturer's user manual for proper use and algorithms.

Choosing an Interface: Nasal vs. Full Face Masks

Interface	Advantages	Disadvantages	Sizing*
Nasal Mask	Comfort Patient compliance	Gas leaks Nasal dryness or damage Normally less efficient ventilation Not usually used for patients in acute respiratory failure Less effective for mouth-breathers	Choose a small mask over a large mask in most cases The top of the mask should be 1/3 of the way down from the bridge of the nose (too high = leaks in eyes) The bottom of the mask should rest just above the upper lip
Full Face Mask	Better ventilation Good seal	More claustrophobic Less patient tolerance Regurgitation and aspiration susceptibility Must remove to expectorate, eat, or speak	Choose a small mask over a large mask, in most cases The top of the mask should be 1/3 of the way down form the bridge of the nose The bottom of the mask should rest just below the lower lip

* See mask manufacturer's instructions for fitting details.

Make It Your Own

Notes Page

10 Diseases and Disorders

CONTENTS

Acute Respiratory Distress Syndrome (ARDS) 10-2
Asthma 10-13
Asthma (Near Fatal) 10-17
Bronchopleural Fistula (B-P Fistula) 10-19
Burns and Smoke Inhalation 10-21
Chronic Obstructive Pulmonary Disease 10-23
Cardiac (MI and CHF) 10-26
Drug Overdose 10-29
Neuromuscular Disorders 10-30
Post-Operative Patients 10-32
Restrictive Pulmonary Lung Disease 10-34
Trauma (Chest) 10-35
Trauma (Head) 10-37

This chapter is meant to discuss noninvasive and invasive ventilator strategies related to specific diseases and disorders. You can find more complete information in Oakes' Clinical Practitioner's Pocket Guide, at RespiratoryUpdate.com, and extensive critical care management in Oakes' Critical Care Pocket Guide.

In most cases, recommendations on specific modes of ventilation are suggestions only, with a lack of definitive evidence on one mode over another. Ultimately it comes down to the critical thinking of the clinician being far more important than the name of any certain mode!

Acute Respiratory Distress Syndrome (ARDS)

An acute, diffuse, inflammatory lung injury resulting in diminished Functional Residual Capacity (FRC), severe shunting, alveolar transudates, ↓ surfactant (washout) atelectasis, ↓ compliance, and severe hypoxemia.

A note about defining:

ARDS went through a definition clarification in 2013 and is now referred to as the "Berlin definition". The "old" definition differentiated acute lung injury (ALI), which has now morphed into Mild, Moderate, and Severe ARDS.

Diagnostic Criteria:

1. **Acute Onset of Respiratory Distress**
   Must be within 7 days of a defined event (sepsis, trauma, pneumonia, etc.). Most cases occur within 72 hours

2. **Hypoxemia:**

Severity of ARDS	PaO_2/FIO_2 ratio (P/F)
Mild	200 - 300
Moderate	100 - 200
Severe	< 100

3. **Bilateral consolidation on CXR or CT**
   Diffuse bilateral infiltates (consistent with pulmonary edema)

4. **Ruled out cardiac failure and fluid overload**
   Determined either by PCWP < 18 cmH_2O (noncardiogenic), or by clinical examination (Because PA Catheters are less common, examination techniques, such as echocardiography, are now seen as acceptable)

Phases

Phase 1 (first 7-10 days) Exudative
Intense inflammatory response resulting in: 1) Alveolar and endothelial damage 2) Increased vascular permeability (= pulmonary edema) 3) Increased water and protein 4) Some component of pulmonary hypertension
Phase 2 (10+ days) Fibroproliferative
Extensive pulmonary fibrosis, which usually resolves (acute fibrosis resolves, though some residual fibrosis may remain)

Clinical Presentation

Clinical features of ARDS usually appear 6-72 hours after an acute event, and progressively worsens:

- Dyspnea
- Tachypnea, Tachycardia
- Acute Respiratory Alkalosis (initial, followed by Respiratory Acidosis as patient begins to tire)
- ↓ C_L (total C < 30 mL/cmH_2O)
- Intrapulmonary shunting (> 20%)
- Marked ↑ in WOB
- PCWP < 15-18 mmHg
- Refractory hypoxemia ($PaO_2/FiO_2 \leq 300$)
- Chest X-ray (bilateral alveolar infiltrates)

Visit **RespiratoryUpdate.com** for further information on ARDS, including a more in-depth discussion of changes in the definition, causes of ARDS, etc.

Ventilator Strategies:

Noninvasive

Consider a TRIAL* of NPPV potentially if:

- Hemodynamically stable
- Able to tolerate a face mask and settings
- Able to maintain a patent airway

*If patient fails to show improvement after a brief trial, consider invasive ventilation

Invasive

- Little evidence exists to definitely recommend Pressure or Volume ventilation, and neither has any one mode been definitively proven to be superior over another.
- The recommendation is that whatever is utilized, the clinician should pay careful attention to preventing further lung injury (in other words: utilize lung protective strategies), providing adequate support, and maintaining adequate oxygenation (note this is different than normal oxygenation).

Notes on Volume Ventilation:

- The ARDS lung is not uniformly injured. Some portions of the affected lung have ↓ C whereas other regions may retain a more normal C. Most of the V_T of a positive pressure breath is delivered to the regions of better C, resulting in over-distension of the more normal lung tissue and causing ventilator-induced lung injury (VILI). For these reasons, V_T should be kept as low as possible.
- In Volume Ventilation, a decelerating flow pattern is often recommended to deliver the majority of V_T early in the inspiratory phase in order to minimize the difference between peak Paw and peak P_{alv}.

Initial Ventilator Settings

Mode	Lung protective (exact mode is less important than lung protective strategy) Consider aggressive lung protection (APRV, HFOV, etc.) early in ARDS progression.
V_T	Starting V_T no greater than 8 cc/kg IBW
f	12-20/min (permissive hypercapnia is acceptable) *Note*: V_T and *f* are selected to minimize P_{alv} and auto-PEEP. ↑ *f* to maintain $\dot{V}_E$ as V_T is ↓
T_I	0.8 - 1.2 sec *Note*: lengthen T_I to improve oxygenation only after V_T, *f* and PEEP have been optimized. ↑ in 0.1 sec increments to achieve oxygenation target (rather than a specific I:E ratio)
T_E	Allow adequate T_E to avoid auto-PEEP
F_IO_2	As needed to achieve PaO_2 target (~ 60 torr)
$\overline{P}aw$	Lowest level to achieve PaO_2 target while maintaining hemodynamic stability (vasopressor support may be necessary)
P_{plat}	Keep ≤ 30 cmH_20 (permissive hypercapnia is allowed)
PEEP	Higher PEEP strategies are recommended, particularly due to presence of pulmonary edema *(the pressure helps drive fluid from lungs and thus improve V/Q). PEEP should be set using optimal PEEP techniques (see Optimal PEEP)*

Key Management Strategies

All management is aimed at preventing lung injury while maintaining minimally adequate oxygenation and ventilation. The clinician is supporting the patient while the ARDS inflammatory process works itself through.

Ventilation

- ↓ V_T to as low as 4 cc/kg when P_{alv} > 30 cmH_2O.
- Palv > 30 cmH_2O may be acceptable in conditions with ↓ Ccw.

Lung recruitment (See Ventilator Management Chapter)

- To date there is inusfficient evidence to support the routine use of recruitment maneuvers with ARDS (particularly with mortality). Due to the heterogenous population, it is possible that some ARDS patients may benefit from recruitment techniques.

PEEP

- Current recommended levels to maintain lung recruitment involve either optimization (see Optimal PEEP), or generally:

Mild ARDS:	8-15 cmH_2O
Moderate-Severe ARDS:	10-20 cmH_2O

See also the PEEP/F_IO_2 tables in the ARDSnet protocol (though there is some controversy surrounding the use of the tables)

Sedation/Paralysis

- The need for sedation varies by patient and strategy. Some strategies, such as APRV require minimal sedation while other strategies, like HFOV require maximal sedation and possible use of neuromuscular blockade (paralytics).

Arterial Blood Gas Management

PaO_2:	Mild ARDS ≥ 70 mmHg Moderate ARDS ≥ 60 mmHg Severe ARDS ≥ 55 mmHg	**pH:** > 7.15 **$PaCO_2$:** (Intentional Hypercapnia)

Permissive hypercapnia ($PaCO_2$ < 100 mmHg) is permissible to limit Palv ≤ 30 cmH_2O. It is usually a necessity once auto-PEEP develops (unless contraindicated or ↑ ICP).

Weaning

- Once improvement in oxygenation occurs, weaning can be considered.
- No one weaning attempt has been proven superior over any other. See ARDSnet guidelines in pages following for more details.

Alternative Techniques for ARDS

High Frequency Ventilation (Oscillator)	Somewhat controversial in light of current evidence-based medicine (see RespiratoryUpdate.com for more details)
inhaled Nitric Oxide (iNO)	Controversial: May be useful in severe life-threatening ARDS (due to Pulmonary Hypertension component)
Inverse Ratio Ventilation	Complicated management due to higher risk of air trapping
Extra-Corporeal Membrane Oxygenation (ECMO)	VV ECMO may be beneficial (allows lungs to rest, preventing injury)
Prone Positioning	Data is inconsistent on effect on morbidity and mortality

ARDSnet PROTOCOL Information

ACUTE PHASE

Relationship between PEEP and F_iO_2 Settings in the ARDS Net Protocol

Low PEEP Approach		High PEEP Approach**	
F_iO_2	PEEP	F_iO_2	PEEP
0.3	5	0.3	12
0.4	5	0.3	14
0.4	8	0.4	14
0.5	8	0.4	16
0.5	10	0.5	16
0.6	10	0.5	18
0.7	10	0.5-0.8	20
0.7	12	0.8	22
0.7	14	0.9	22
0.8	14	1.0	22-24
0.9	14		
0.9	16		
0.9	18		
1.0	18		
1.0	20-24		
1.0	26-34*		

F_iO_2 and/or PEEP are adjusted in intervals of 5-15 mins until values are compatible with the table. As PEEP is increased, P_{plat} is re-measured to see if V_T is to be reduced below 6 cc/kg.

*When PaO_2 < 55 mmHg or SpO_2 < 88% on F_iO_2 1.0 and PEEP = 24 cmH_2O, then I:E is ↑ to 1:1 and PEEP is ↑ in increments of 2 cmH_2O until a maximum of 34 cmH_2O or until PaO_2 > 55 mmHg or SpO_2 > 88%. If no improvement occurs by 4 hrs, then PEEP is ↓ to 24 cmH_2O.

NHLBI ARDS Clinical Trials Network. Higher versus lower positive end-expiratory pressures in patients with the acute respiratory distress syndrom. ***N Engl J Med* 351: 327-336, 2004

Protocol Ranges: PaO_2 55 – 80 mmHg, SpO_2 88 – 95%

Note: Mild hypoxemia is preferred over high levels of F_iO_2 and PEEP. Promptly ↓ F_iO_2 and PEEP levels when upper levels are reached.

In the presence of severe hypoxemia or severe acidosis:
Pplat limit of 30 cmH_2O may be temporarily suspended.

When severe patient-ventilator asynchrony occurs:
V_T may be ↑ to 7 - 8 mL/kg as long as Pplat ≤ 30 cmH_2O.
Set *f* is adjusted between 6 - 35 breaths/min to maintain pH 7.30 – 7.45. High levels of sedation are often necessary to control the restlessness and anxiety associated with low V_T and/or hypercapnia.

ARDS NET Protocol Adjustments

Condition	Recommended Adjustment
P_{plat} > 30 cmH_20	↓ V_T by 1 cc/kg every 2-3 hr, down to a minimum of 4 cc/kg ↑ f to maintain $\dot{V}_E$
Pplat < 25 cmH_20 and V_T < 6 mL/kg	↑ V_T to 6 cc/kg and ↓ f to maintain $\dot{V}_E$
Mild Acidosis: pH 7.15-7.30	↑ f to 35 breaths/min or until pH ≥ 7.30 with $PaCO_2$ ≥ 25 mm Hg. If pH remains < 7.30 and $PaCO_2$ < 25 mmHg, consider treatment with $NaHCO_3$.
Severe Acidosis: pH < 7.15	↑ f to 35 breaths/min and consider treatment of pH with $NaHCO_3$. If pH remains < 7.15, ↑ V_T by 1 cc/kg until pH > 7.15. Pplat > 30 cmH_2O is acceptable Upper limits of V_T and Pplat are suspended until pH = 7.20.
Severe Hypoxemia: PaO_2 < 55 mm Hg (SpO_2 < 88%) on F_IO_2 1.0 and PEEP 24 cmH_2O	Upper limits of V_T and P_{plat} are suspended during PEEP trial between 26 and 34 cmH_2O. I:E is set at 1:1
Severe Patient-Ventilator dyssynchrony: The failure of the ventilator to pressurize the circuit above PEEP during inspiration, or double-triggering the ventilator during inspiration (> 3/min).	↑ f and ↓ I:E to ↑ $\dot{V}_I$ Maximize trigger sensitivity If available on VV, use decelerating flow pattern to ↑ $\dot{V}_I$. If above measures ineffective and Pplat < 30 cmH_2O, ↑ V_T by 1 cc/kg up to 8 cc.

Monitor Hemo Status Closely: response to low V_T ventilation (including hypercapnia, respiratory acidosis, sedation, low V_T, high PEEP, patient's underlying disease, etc.) is complex and varied.

Low V_T ventilation is disadvantageous to pulmonary hygiene and ↑ the risk of retained secretions. Adequate humidification is essential and transient hyperinflation to promote secretion clearance (esp. with suctioning or CPT) should be considered when secretions are thick.

Recovery Phase (Weaning Protocol)

Two ARDS Network Weaning Protocol Algorithms:

1) **Overview**
2) **Weaning from A/C Ventilation to Unassisted Breathing**

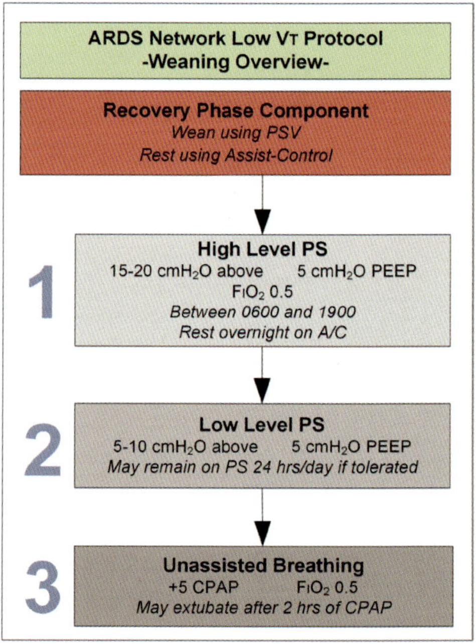

Algorithms on this page and next, adapted from Kallet RH, Corral W, Silverman HJ, Luce JM. Implementation of a Low Tidal Volume Ventilation Protocol for Patients with Acute Lung Injury or Acute Respiratory Distress Syndrome. ***Resp Care*** 2001; 46(10): 1024-1037

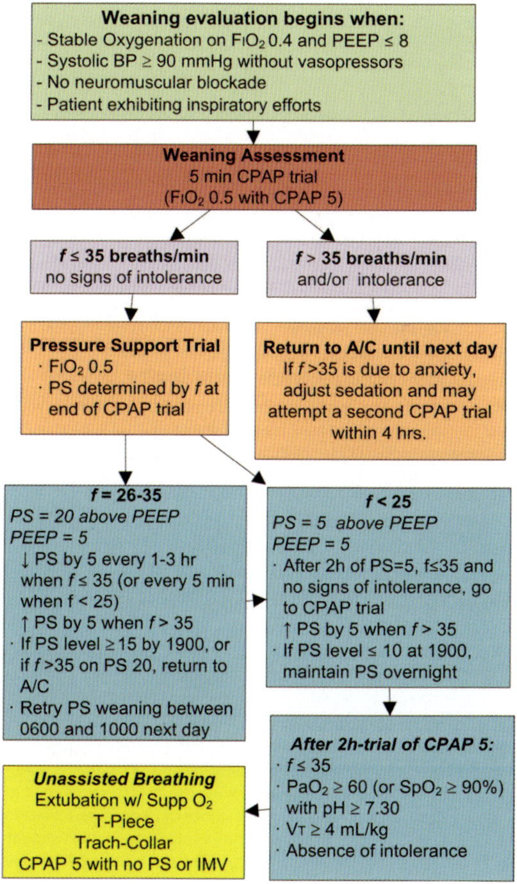
Weaning evaluation begins when:
- Stable Oxygenation on F_IO_2 0.4 and PEEP ≤ 8
- Systolic BP ≥ 90 mmHg without vasopressors
- No neuromuscular blockade
- Patient exhibiting inspiratory efforts
Weaning Assessment
5 min CPAP trial
(F_IO_2 0.5 with CPAP 5)
f ≤ 35 breaths/min
no signs of intolerance
f > 35 breaths/min
and/or intolerance
Pressure Support Trial
· F_IO_2 0.5
· PS determined by f at end of CPAP trial
Return to A/C until next day
If f >35 is due to anxiety, adjust sedation and may attempt a second CPAP trial within 4 hrs.
f = 26-35
PS = 20 above PEEP
PEEP = 5
↓ PS by 5 every 1-3 hr when f ≤ 35 (or every 5 min when f < 25)
↑ PS by 5 when f > 35
· If PS level ≥ 15 by 1900, or if f >35 on PS 20, return to A/C
· Retry PS weaning between 0600 and 1000 next day
f < 25
PS = 5 above PEEP
PEEP = 5
· After 2h of PS=5, f≤35 and no signs of intolerance, go to CPAP trial
↑ PS by 5 when f > 35
· If PS level ≤ 10 at 1900, maintain PS overnight
After 2h-trial of CPAP 5:
· f ≤ 35
· PaO_2 ≥ 60 (or SpO_2 ≥ 90%) with pH ≥ 7.30
· V_T ≥ 4 mL/kg
· Absence of intolerance
Unassisted Breathing
Extubation w/ Supp O_2
T-Piece
Trach-Collar
CPAP 5 with no PS or IMV

Clinical Notes

- F_IO_2 and PEEP have either ↓ or remained stable during previous day. Dopamine or dobutamine infusions of ≤ 5 µg/kg/min are not considered vasopressor support.
- Evaluate for weaning between 6:00 and 10:00 AM
- If patient is not triggering breaths, reduce mandatory *f* by 50% for 5 min. If still no triggering, then patient does not meet weaning criteria. (May re-evaluate after any sedation is ↓).

Criteria Used to Assess Weaning Tolerance

Total *f* ≤ 35 breaths/min (>35 breaths/min for ≤ 5 min is allowed)
SpO_2 ≥ 88% (< 88% for < 15 min is allowed)
No respiratory distress, defined as <u>*2 or more*</u> of the following:

- HR > 120% of 6:00 AM value (> 120% for 5 min is allowed)
- Pronounced accessory muscle use
- Abdominal paradox
- Diaphoresis
- Pronounced subjective sense of dyspnea

↑ Raw – bronchospasm and mucosal edema with ↑ secretions resulting in ball-valving and long time-constants
Air-trapping (auto-PEEP) – ↑ FRC and ↓ CL resulting in ↑ WOB and barotrauma
Large intrathoracic pressure changes – resulting in altered gas distribution and altered perfusion
Progressive hypoxemia and anxiety

Indications for Mechanical Ventilation

Acute respiratory failure Air-trapping on CXR BS absent and chest hyperresonant to percussion Exhaustion (↑ or ↓ RR and altered consciousness)	Impending respiratory failure (rising $PaCO_2$ and falling pH) Life threatening arrhythmias Respiratory or cardiac arrest Severe refractory hypoxemia

Clinical Note: The respiratory distress in these patients is generally due to hypoxemia, which in turn results in hypocarbia ($PaCO_2$ < 40 mm Hg). MV is generally instituted when the $PaCO_2$ climbs back to normal (40 mmHg), which is now indicative of impending respiratory failure due to fatigue. At this point, full ventilatory support should not be delayed because severe hypercarbia and acidosis will develop rapidly.

Asthma

Careful consideration should be given to preventing invasive ventilation of patients with Asthma when possible. However, once a patient is deemed to be in failure, any delay in intubation should be avoided.

Patient Problems:

- ↑ Raw: Bronchospasm and mucosal edema with ↑ secretions which may result in "ball-valving" and long time constants
- Auto PEEP: ↑ Functional Residual Capacity and ↓ Compliance, which results in ↑ WOB and risk of barotrauma
- Large intrathoracic pressure changes: result in altered gas distribution and altered perfusion
- Progressive hypoxemia and anxiety

Indications for Ventilator Support

- Acute respiratory failure*
- Hyperexpansion on CXR
- Diminished air flow on auscultation (or absent)
- Exhaustion (↑ or ↓ RR and altered consciousness)
- Life-threatening dysrhythmias
- Respiratory/Cardiac Arrest
- Severe refractory hypoxemia

**ABG will likely start as Respiratory Alkalosis, but then appear to normalize as patient tires (pH/$PaCO_2$ will normalize with underlying hypoxemia), before finally resulting in Respiratory Acidosis.* Patients should be considered for intubation when $PaCO_2$ and pH appear normal (in context).

Disease Management

Type of Ventilation

Although no one type of ventilation is superior, patients generally don't tolerate assisted ventilation, and PV is commonly preferred for severe asthma. Advantages of PV: A change in V_T is a good indicator of change in resistance and air-trapping, T_I is not prematurely terminated by a high pressure limit, and flow will adjust automatically.

Noninvasive

Use of NPPV is controversial but may support a patient's ventilatory needs for a short trial (to allow time for steroids and bronchodilators to become effective)

Limitations of NPPV:

- Increases risk of aspiration
- May cause heightened sense of air hunger
- High risk of auto-PEEP

Initial Settings:

When $F_IO_2 < 0.70$ / $PaCO_2 < 50$ mmHg:

CPAP	Start at 5 cmH_2O and titrate for SpO_2
F_IO_2	1.0, then wean as clinically indicated

When $F_IO_2 > 0.70$ / $PaCO_2 > 50$ mmHg

BiPAP	start at IPAP 8-10 / EPAP 3-5 Titrate up to 10-12 / 5-7 Maintain ΔP (IPAP - EPAP) of at least 5 cmH_2O
F_IO_2	1.0, then wean as clinically indicated

Invasive

Do not delay intubation once determined to be necessary:

- Lack of improvement or increased WOB on NPPV
- Persistent hypercapnia ($PaCO_2$ > 50 mmHg)
- Refractory hypoxemia (F_IO_2 > 0.60)
- Altered mental status

Caution: manipulation of the airway may cause increased obstruction due to exaggerated bronchial responsiveness

When manually ventilating pay close attention to allowing for adequate T_E.

Mode	Pressure ventilation is commonly preferred: • changing V_T is a good indicator of change in Raw and auto-PEEP • T_I is not prematurely terminated by a high pressure limit • Flow is variable/automatic
V_T	Starting V_T 6-8 cc/kg IBW Decrease V_T to keep PIP < 40 and Pplat < 30
f	Lower Rates (8-12 breaths/min) Rationale: Prevent auto-PEEP
T_I	0.75 - 1.2 sec Verify T_E is adequate for exhalation (use flow scalar or measure auto-PEEP) High $\dot{V}_I$ (80 - 100 L/min) I:E of 1:3 to 1:5
F_IO_2	Wean for SpO_2 > 92%
PEEP	3-8 cmH_2O, then titrate as needed

- Monitor closely for auto-PEEP with any ventilator or patient status changes.
- Certainly consider in-line continuous bronchodilators and/or other adjuncts such as Heliox delivery (if ventilator calibrated appropriately).

National Asthma Education Guidelines*

Signs of Impending Respiratory Failure:

Altered mental state
Worsening fatigue
$PaCO_2 \geq 42$

Intubation: DO NOT DELAY ONCE DEEMED NECESSARY (see Near-Fatal Asthma below for intubation indications and procedure.)

Heliox (Heliox-driven Albuterol treatments) or $MgSO_4$ may be considered to avoid intubation.

Mechanical Ventilation - Initial Settings

V_T	6 - 10 mL/kg (VV) (↓ V_T to keep PIP < 35 cmH_2O)
PV:	keep PIP ≤ 30 - 35 cmH_2O
f	12 – 25 breaths/min
PEEP	4 - 10 cm H_2O
F_IO_2	1.0
T_I	Keep short enough to ensure expiration ends before next inspiration.

Clinical Notes: Immediately assess for chest rise, BS, airflow, and T_E. Monitor for auto-PEEP and barotrauma. Monitor with end-tidal CO_2

Permissive hypercapnia is the recommended strategy, but it is not uniformly successful. Minimize high airway pressures and barotrauma.

*Adapted from the ***Guidelines for the Diagnosis and Management of Asthma, the National Asthma Education Program's Expert Panel: Report 2, 1998, and EPR-3, 2007***; National Heart Lung, and Blood Institute; National Institutes of Health, Bethesda, MD.

Near-Fatal Asthma

Sometimes referred to as "Status Asthmaticus".

Noninvasive

A very brief trial of NPPV could be considered, though the patient is unlikely to succeed if truly in a near-fatal state. This requires clinical judgment.

Invasive

Indications:

- Apnea
- Obtunded/Comatose or Severe Agitation/Distress
- Exhaustion
- Diaphoresis (severe)
- Lack of muscle tone
- Clearly worsening Respiratory Acidosis

Procedure:

- RSI is recommended with the largest ET Tube clinically indicated (decreases Raw)
- Consider instilling albuterol (2.5 - 5.0 mg) post-intubation

Mode	Pressure ventilation is commonly preferred: changing V_T is a good indicator of change in Raw and auto-PEEP
V_T	6-8 cc/kg IBW
f	6-10 breaths/min
Flow ($\dot{V}_I$)	80 - 100 L/min with decelerating pattern

Disease Management

Troubleshooting: Hypotension or Desaturation After Intubating

Check for tension pneumothorax:

- Check for: 1) Unilateral chest expansion; 2) tracheal shift; 3) subcutaneous emphysema (crepitus)
- Decompression – insert 16 gauge needle into 2nd IC space, mid-clavicular line. Insert chest tube if air is emitted.

Check and treat auto-PEEP

(the most common cause of profound hypotension)

Consider:

- Stop ventilation for < 1 min to allow auto-PEEP to dissipate.
- Decrease inhalation time (increasing exhalation indirectly)
- Decrease *f* by 2 breaths/min at a time
- Decrease V_T down to 3-5 cc/kg IBW
- Observe oxygenation.

Bronchoconstriction

Intubation and Ventilation can trigger further bronchoconstriction Consider continuous bronchodilators and possibly Heliox administration during ventilation

If airway is difficult to ventilate, perform the following, in order, until ventilation is adequate: ‡

1) Ensure passive patient-ventilator interaction (sedated or paralyzed).
2) Check ET tube for patency.
3) Ensure adequate V_T: ↑ T_E, ↓T_I and ↑ PIP
4) ↓ Rate to 6 - 8/min (to ↓ auto-PEEP to ≤ 15 cmH_2O)
5) ↓ V_T to 3 - 5 cc/kg (to ↓ auto-PEEP to ≤ 15 cmH_2O).
6) ↑ $\dot{V}_I$ to > 60 L/min (may use 90 - 120 LPM to further shorten T_I and ↑ I:E ratio).

Monitoring

Careful monitoring for auto-PEEP & barotrauma (P_{plat}, $\overline{P}aw$, V_T)

‡ Brief Synopsis of the Guidelines 2000 for Cardiopulmonary Resuscitation and Emergency Cardiovascular Care: International Consensus on Science. AHA and the International Liaison Committee of Resuscitation, Circulation, 2000; 102 (Suppl I): I-1-384, and 2005 Update; Circulation, 2005, Vol 112, No. 24; Circulation, 2010

Bronchopleural (B-P) Fistula

A "hole" between the bronchial tree and the pleural space, this can be caused by trauma, surgery, invasive procedures or certain diffuse lung disease processes.

Type of Ventilation

- No single mode or approach has been shown more effective
- A ventilator capable of delivering high $\dot{V}_I$ and large V_T may be required when a large air leak is present
- PV is often recommended due to the ability to control peak P_{alv}.
- Avoid PSV IF B-P fistula leak is > than the flow level required to terminate inspiration, then the ventilator will not cycle from I to E
- Minimize the number of full ventilator-delivered breaths (PSV or low rate SIMV)
- Minimize pressures and T_I
- Allowing spontaneous ventilation is dependent on the severity of the disease and patient hemodynamics

Note: Non-conventional approaches include ILV and HFV. Neither have been shown to improve outcome.

Mode	Pressure ventilation is commonly preferred: changing V_T is a good indicator of change in Raw and auto-PEEP
V_T	4-8 cc/kg IBW
f	10-30 breaths/min (depends on underlying process)
Flow ($\dot{V}_I$)	70 - 100 L/min with decelerating pattern
PEEP	0 - 10 cmH_2O (minimize when possible)

Indication for Mechanical Ventilation

B-P fistula in itself is not an indication for MV. Rather, its presence is often in conjunction with other pulmonary problems.

Key Management Strategies

- The goal is to minimize inflation pressures and V_T.
- Use a mode that minimizes transpulmonary pressures (PIP, P_{alv}, PEEP) to minimize air leak through the fistula.
  - Minimize T_I, PIP, Pplat, PEEP when possible
  - Minimize chest tube suction (may trigger ventilator)
- Use the lowest V_T that allows adequate ventilation.
- Ventilatory support should provide adequate inflation for the uninvolved areas of lung.
- Consider permissive hypercapnia to minimize inspiratory pressures and volumes.

Note: The flow through a fistula is proportional to the magnitude and duration of the pressure gradient (e.g., Palv 30 cmH_2O and chest tube suction - 20 cmH_2O = 50 cmH_2O pressure gradient).

Management of oxygenation is often difficult because most maneuvers which ↑ PaO_2 (↑ PEEP, ↑ $\overline{P}aw$, ↑ T_I) also ↑ leak.

Consider ILV or HFV in cases of severe leak.

Monitoring

- Careful monitoring of pressures and the volume of air leak (inspired V_T - expired V_T).

Weaning

- Weaning strategy is based on the underlying disease process and closure of the air leak.

Burns and Smoke Inhalation

Includes: 1. Surface Burns (causes restriction)
2. Inhalation (Thermal, Parenchymal, Toxic)

Complications Associated with Burns and Smoke Inhalation:

- ARDS
- Airway obstruction
- CO poison
- Pneumonia
- Pulmonary edema
- Pulmonary embolism
- Sepsis
- Upper airway/ bronchial obstruction

Noninvasive

- NPPV is relatively contraindicated for burns. It may be an acceptable delivery device in Carbon Monoxide poisoning, but only if there are no concerns with LOC.

Invasive

Indications for Mechanical Ventilation

Surface Burns:	***Thermal Injury:***
ARDS due to sepsis, or hyper-metabolism. Chest restriction due to severe burns. Respiratory depression from pain medication.	Most common effects are upper airway edema, spasm, and ↑ secretions. Immediate intubation is indicated due to risk of complete airway obstruction. MV may not be required if there is no lower airway injury.
Parenchymal Injury:	***Systemic Toxins:***
Smoke inhalation induces bronchospasm and ↓ mucociliary transport. These patients commonly develop ARDS (see ARDS section).	Respiratory depression due to CO poisoning, cyanide, and/or nitrogen oxides.

Type of Ventilation

No one type of ventilation has been proven to be superior over another with burns/inhalation. An argument for Pressure may be made if ↑ Raw or ↓ CL. Full ventilatory support is often required, at least initially.

V_T	6-8 cc/kg IBW
f	15-25 breaths/min (lower if auto-PEEP)
TI	1.0 second or less
PEEP	5 cmH_2O (start)
F_IO_2	1.0 (especially in presence of carbon monoxide)

Key Management Strategies

- Many patients require sedation and paralysis.
- If patient develops ARDS, see ARDS section.
- Patients who are hypermetabolic may require high $\dot{V}_E$ to maintain normocarbia.
- PaO_2 is often normal or ↑, but an F_IO_2 of 1.0 is mandatory for the treatment of CO poison until the measured carboxyhemoglobin level is < 10%. Hyperbaric O_2 therapy is useful if available.

Monitoring

- Pulse oximetry may be unreliable if a high carboxyhemoglobin level is present.
- Closely monitor for auto-PEEP if high $\dot{V}_E$ is used or patient exhibits bronchospasm and/or ↑ secretions.

Weaning

- Reversal of the acute process usually leads to early and quick weaning, provided there are no secondary complications, such as ARDS, sepsis, or pulmonary infections.

Chronic Obstructive Pulmonary Disease (COPD) (Exacerbations)

Much thought must be given by the clinical team as to how to best address COPD exacerbations, with most clinicians preferring aggressive trials of NPPV (unless contraindicated) over invasive ventilation where weaning can become problematic (accessory muscles, required for baseline breathing in these patients, have potentially atrophied).

Noninvasive

- As stated above, NPPV should be considered as a first option for most patients in acute exacerbation. Invasive ventilation strategies may be associated with increased morbidity.

Selection and Exclusion Criteria for NPPV †

Indications for trialing NPPV (*at least 1*):

1. **Respiratory Acidosis**: pH < 7.35 and/or ≥ $PaCO_2$ 45 mmHg
2. **Severe dyspnea** with clinical signs of:
   - Respiratory muscle fatigue and/or ↑ WOB:
     - Accessory muscle use
     - Paradoxical abdominal motion
     - Intercostal retractions

Contraindications (When NOT to use NPPV):

- See NPPV Chapter for general contraindications to NPPV. In addition care should be used with patients with known bullous emphysema

BiPAP	Start at IPAP 8-10 / EPAP 3-5 Titrate by V_T and alleviation of WOB Maintain ΔP (IPAP - EPAP) of at least 5 cmH_2O
F_IO_2	Dependent on severity of COPD, titrate to desired SpO_2/PaO_2

Disease Management

Invasive

Indications (in addition to general indications for intubation):

- Failure on trial of noninvasive (NPPV)
- Lack of tolerance of NPPV
- pH < 7.25 and $PaCO_2$ > 60 mmHg (note that $PaCO_2$ should not be interpreted apart from the pH)

Type of Ventilation

While no evidence supports any particular mode over another, some clinicians choose pressure modes (A/C or PSV) because:

- Flow-on-demand to meet patient's needs
- Set T_I
- back up rate
- patient triggering allowed.

Full ventilatory support is recommended for the first 24-48 hrs because most patients are completely exhausted after several days of ↑ WOB.

V_T	6-8 cc/kg IBW
f	8-16 breaths/min (allows for maximal exhalation, and prevents air trapping)
T_I	0.6 - 1.2 sec (allows for maximal exhalation) Resulting I:E ratio 1:4 - 1:6 as needed
PEEP	5 cmH_2O (start) May consider PEEP to match 80% of measured auto-PEEP when triggering dyssynchrony noted
F_IO_2	Maintain PaO_2 > 60 mmHg Do not withold oxygen from a patient who is hypoxic
Flow ($\dot{V}_I$)	60 - 100 L/min with decelerating pattern

Do Not Overcorrect acid-base balance (by allowing $PaCO_2$ to get to normal range), but instead target normal pH and consider pateint's baseline, if available.

Key Management Strategies

- ↓ WOB (unload and rest ventilatory muscles)
- ↓ $PaCO_2$ to patient's baseline
- Treat hypoxemia
- Maintain $P_{plat} \leq 30$ cmH_2O. (Permissive hypercapnia is acceptable if needed to keep $P_{alv} < 30$ cmH_2O). *See Chapter 8.*
- ↓ Raw (bronchodilators and corticosteroids)
- Minimize air-trapping and auto-PEEP – use the least $\dot{V}_E$ (↓ V_T and slow *f*) that produces an acceptable gas exchange and the greatest T_E. (Note: ↑ Raw requires a greater T_E to expel all the air).
- Applied PEEP may be helpful to ↓ WOB when auto-PEEP exists.
- Maximize patient-ventilator synchrony.
- ↓ patient anxiety
- Provide adequate secretion hydration, mobilization, and removal.
- Provide adequate nutrition.

Monitoring

Closely monitor for:

- Auto-PEEP (for signs of auto-PEEP see Ventilator Management Chapter).
- Clinical signs of cardiopulmonary distress (RR, BS, retractions, etc)
- Patient-ventilator asynchrony
- Systemic and pulmonary hemodynamic changes (pulse, BP, PAP)

Weaning

To date, there is no definitive best approach. NPPV and weaning protocols have been shown to shorten weaning time

Cardiac (MI and CHF)

Patients who present with CHF exacerbations (pulmonary edema) often respond very well to CPAP noninvasively, usually in amounts greater than physiologic. The idea is that the "highest pressure wins" and fluid is pushed out of the lung parenchyma. MI's are more complicated and require careful clinical judgment as to when to trial NPPV as opposed to when to intubate and allow the workload on the heart to be alleviated.

Patient Problems

- Severe heart failure leads to hypoxemia, ↑ WOB, and ↑ work of myocardium.

Precipitating Causes: Acute MI, fluid overload, ↑ BP, tachycardia with ↓ fill time, valve disease.

Noninvasive

- Patients who present with pulmonary edema, including flash pulmonary edema (which can appear emergent) often respond well to CPAP via mask. The sooner the CPAP is initiated, the more successful it is likely to be.

Initial NPPV Settings

CPAP	5-15 cmH_2O (usually 10-15 is required)
F_IO_2	1.0

- The use of NPPV with MI is more controversial as any dyssynchrony/intolerance of NPPV will likely add to the workload of the heart during a time when this may not be tolerated

Invasive

- In the presence of myocardial ischemia, choose modes that ↓ WOB.
- Modes that ↑ WOB will ↑ O_2 demand and detrimentally affect myocardial O_2 supply and demand.
- Spontaneous ventilation in patients with myocardial ischemia and high lung resistance and/or poor respiratory muscle function is likely detrimental.
- Full ventilatory support with F_IO_2 of 1.0 is recommended initially, until ABG data is obtained to support weaning.

Initial Ventilator Settings

V_T	6-8 cc/kg IBW
f	≥ 15 breaths/min
TI	≤ 1 sec
Flow ($\dot{V}_I$)	> 60 L/min with decelerating pattern
PEEP	5-10 cmH_2O (monitor hemodynamics carefully)
F_IO_2	1.0

Key Management Strategies

Select a mode of ventilation that minimizes WOB.

Consider the potentially beneficial effects* of PPV on decreasing venous return and improving oxygenation in patients with severe CHF and life-threatening hypoxemia.

*PPV and PEEP may have variable effects on myocardial function and oxygenation depending on whether the LV is normal or failing.

Monitoring

- Careful monitoring and assessment of the effects of PPV on hemodynamics, as well as fluid and electrolyte balance is essential.

Weaning

- Any technique is suitable, though care with any PEEP titration should be used.
- The process is dependent on any underlying pulmonary problems.
- Caution with PEEP titration because of complex effects on myocardial function.
- CV function can change dramatically as intrathoracic pressure changes with the withdrawal of PPV and PEEP, especially the LV preload and potential pulmonary edema. The removal of PEEP is usually one of the last steps in the process.
- Fluid balance and inotropes must be titrated concurrently to ensure maximum myocardial contractility.

Cardiac Surgery (CABG, etc.)

- Patients often arrive from surgery sedated and possibly paralyzed. Hemodynamics are closely monitored, but many of these patients are rapidly weaned with aggressive goals to extubate (within hours) post-CABG.

CABG = Coronary Artery Bypass Graft

Drug Overdose

Not all drug overdoses result in intubation, but patients should be assessed closely and if obtunded, with respiratory depression, or with any CV compromise, INVASIVE ventilation should be considered. **For the most part NPPV is contraindicated.**

Invasive

Type of Ventilation

Any type that supports ventilation is acceptable.

Initial Ventilator Settings

V_T	6-8 cc/kg IBW
f	15-20 breaths/min
TI	Normal
PEEP	5 cmH_2O (to maintain FRC)
F_IO_2	Minimal F_IO_2 is usually required unless patient aspirated in addition to the overdose

Monitoring

Monitor closely for:

- Aspiration, hemodynamic stability, LOC, patient-vent synchrony

Weaning

- Discontinuation is indicated when the drug is cleared and adequate spontaneous ventilation is restored.

Underlying drug addiction or ETOH history may significantly complicate synchrony and weaning. There is no easy "one size fits all" strategy for working with these patients.

Neuromuscular Disorders

Key problems requiring attention are often related to airway patency (aspiration), impaired mucociliary clearance, and atelectasis (inadequate ventilation).

Two Types

Rapid Onset (days to weeks)	Gradual Onset (months to years)
Botulism	ALS
Cervical spinal cord injury	Muscular dystrophy
Guillian Barré	Post polio syndrome
Myasthenia gravis	Progressive thoracic deformities (scoliosis, kyphosis, kyphoscoliosis)
Poliomyelitis	
Tetanus	

Indication for Mechanical Ventilation

Progressive ventilatory muscle weakness leading to acute respiratory failure. Monitor lung mechanics (NIF, FVC) closely and intubate proactively when patient shows impending failure.

Noninvasive

- NPPV may be preferred in many cases, particularly in acute care when lung volumes are normal. Settings should focus on improving FRC (increased EPAP while maintaining adequate ΔP [IPAP-EPAP])
- Titrate V_T to goal (6-8 cc/kg IBW)
- Of notable concern, patients must be able to protect their own airway adequately to be candidates for NPPV.

Invasive

- There is no evidence that either positive pressure or negative pressure ventilation is superior.
- Full or partial ventilatory support is dependent on the patient's capabilities and disease process.

Initial Ventilator Settings

V_T	Varies but consider lower target V_T (6-8 cc/kg IBW) acutely with consideration for higher V_T at least intermittently (10-15 cc/kg IBW) longer-term
f	Maintain adequate minute ventilation
TI	≤ 1 sec
Flow ($\dot{V}_I$)	≤ 60 L/min (normal lung volumes) ≥ 60 L/min (reduced lung volumes)
PEEP	5 cmH_2O (maintain FRC)
F_IO_2	Should be minimal once lungs are recruited

Key Management Strategies

- The main needs of these patients are adequate lung inflation and aggressive pulmonary hygiene. Provide support based on the patient's inherent ventilatory muscle strengths.
- Psychologically many of these patients desire or demand large V_T, high flow, fast rates, and long T_I (more than needed). Adjust to satisfy patient's inspiratory needs.

Monitoring

- Daily monitoring of spontaneous V_T, *f*, FVC, NIF, and ventilatory pattern. Less frequent ABGs are required.

Weaning

- Primary neuromuscular deficit must be reversed.
- Goal is often independence during the day with support at night.
- Retraining of ventilatory muscles is frequently needed.

Post-Operative Patients

Indications For MV

- Apnea – from unreversed anesthesia (esp. due to hypothermia)
- Complications of phrenic nerve or diaphragmatic injury
- Compromised cardiopulmonary reserve – due to pre-existing lung disease
- Post-op cardiopulmonary stress (esp. heart and lung transplants)
- Post-op pulmonary complications

Noninvasive

- See note in yellow box on next page, but in summary noninvasive ventilation should be considered as a transitional option allowing for earlier extubation in some patients.

Invasive

Initial Ventilator Settings*

V_T	6-8 cc/kg IBW
f	Maintain adequate minute ventilation
TI	Normal Range
PEEP	5 cmH_2O (maintain FRC)
F_IO_2	Titrated to maintain goal PaO_2/SpO2

*These settings are clearly generic, and presume no underlying disease processes

Key Management Strategies

- The greatest concern for the clinician is to avoid healthcare-induced complications of ventilatory support, including infection, ↓ cardiac output, unnecessary sedation, hyperventilation, inspissated secretions, and unnecessary exposure to high F_IO_2.

Monitoring

- Close monitoring of LOC, fluid balance, hemodynamics, and pulmonary mechanics (esp. ability to breathe deeply and cough).

Weaning

- Weaning is commonly quick and easy, but dependent on underlying problems.
- Residual anesthetic effects may require a variable period before weaning is successful.

With all weaning, attention should be paid to pre-existing conditions. In particular, post-op patients should be screened for Obstructive Sleep Apnea (preferably pre-op), and considered for transition from invasive mechanical ventilation to NPPV, as clinically appropriate.

Restrictive Pulmonary Lung Disorders/Diseases

This group of disorders includes thoracic cage abnormalities like kyphoscoliosis; a component of progressive neuromuscular disorders like ALS; and may also include obesity-related syndromes. Severity varies widely.

Noninvasive

- NPPV may successfully treat hypoventilation aspects of these diseases/disorders, particularly as related to respiratory fatigue. Some of these patients manage well during waking hours with no support, but require supplementary support during sleep.
- NPPV should not be considered in any patient who has difficulty managing secretions (airway patency)

Invasive

Similar to COPD except:

V_T	6-8 cc/kg IBW
f	12-30 breaths/min (increased to maintain ↑ $\dot{V}_E$)
TI	≤ 1.0 sec
Flow ($\dot{V}_I$)	≥ 60 L/min with decelerating waveform
PEEP	5 cmH_2O (maintain FRC) Higher PEEP levels may be considered to offset chest wall restrictions, such as with Obesity
F_IO_2	Titrated to maintain goal PaO_2/SpO2

Traumas (Chest)

Types

- Blunt chest trauma
- Penetrating chest trauma

Indications for Ventilation

Blunt Chest Trauma:

<u>*Rib fracture (flail chest)*</u> –

3+ rib fractures suggests need for hospitalization/transfer

Flail chest does not definitively require ventilatory support

Consider invasive ventilation only if the patient also has:

- Deteriorating respiratory status
- Fatigue from WOB
- Compromised lung mechanics
- Respiratory depression secondary to pain control
- Need for immediate surgical intervention
- Shock
- Closed Head Injury

<u>*Pulmonary contusion*</u> – Although clinically similar to ARDS, the localized damage often lends itself to treatment by O_2, CPAP, and positioning. ARDS may develop (treat per ARDS guidelines found elsewhere in this chapter)

Penetrating Chest Trauma

- Ventilatory support is usually post-op.

Type of Ventilation

- NPPV may be considered initially
- Pressure modes may be more appropriate in patients with air leaks and/or barotrauma.
- Full ventilatory support is usually required initially.

Initial Ventilator Settings

V_T	6-8 cc/kg IBW (normal compliance) 4-8 cc/kg IBW (pulmonary contusions)
f	15-25 breaths/min
TI	≤ 1.0 sec
Flow ($\dot{V}_I$)	≥ 60 L/min with decelerating waveform
PEEP	5 cmH_2O (maintain FRC) Use caution with PEEP in presence of air leaks

Key Management Strategies

- Ventilate at the lowest possible mean airway pressures due to risks of pulmonary air leaks (pneumothorax).
- Use PEEP with caution due to barotrauma (esp. unilateral contusion) and hemodynamic instability due to blood loss and/or head injury.
- Many patients require initial sedation, and in rare cases, paralytics.
- Permissive hypercapnia may be employed provided no accompanying head trauma with ↑ ICP.

Monitoring

Monitor closely for signs of:

- Air leak
- Atelectasis
- Pulmonary embolism
- Hemodynamic instability
- Pneumonia (most common complication)

Weaning

- Discontinuation often occurs early and rapidly unless ARDS develops or severe chest wall or diaphragm injury is present.

Traumas (Head)

Types

- Intracerebral Bleeds:
  - Subarachnoid Hemorrhage (SAH)
  - Subdural Hematoma (SDH)
  - Intraventricular Hemorrhage (IVH)
- Diffuse Axonal Injury (DAI)
- Cerebral Contusion
- Concussion

Patient Problems: Cerebral edema and/or ↑ ICP

CPP = MAP – ICP	**CPP > 120** = encephalopathy, cerebral edema
	Normal CPP = 50 - 70
	CPP < 50 = poor perfusion

CPP = Cerebral Perfusion Pressure (mmHg)
MAP = Mean Arterial Pressure (mmHg) ... Normal = 70-80 mmHg
ICP = Intracranial Pressure (mmHg) ... Normal = < 15 mmHg

Common Causes

- Stroke (CVA)
- Hepatic failure
- Post-resuscitation hypoxia
- Surgery (post craniotomy)
- Trauma

Indications for MV

- Central respiratory depression from injury or drugs used to treat acute head injury (barbituate coma, sedation, paralysis)
- Glascow Coma Score (GCS) < 8
- Impending or actual cardiac arrest
- Neurogenic pulmonary edema

Type of Ventilation

- Either volume or pressure ventilation can be used.
- Full ventilatory support should be used initially

Initial Ventilator Settings

V_T	6-8 cc/kg IBW
f	10-15 breaths/min (up to 15-20 for hyperventilation - see below)
TI	≤ 1.0 sec
Flow ($\dot{V}_I$)	High (keep T_I short) with decelerating waveform
PEEP	5 cmH_2O (watch closely) *usually maintained lower than average*
F_IO_2	Use 1.0 initially. Maintain PaO_2 80-100 mmHg (avoids hypoxemia and minimizes ICP increase)

Key Management Strategies

- Patients with head injury are at ↑ risk of aspiration (patency)
- Maintain patient's head in neutral position and 30° elevation
- Maintain normal CPP by maintaining normal MAP + normal ICP

Recommendations (Brain Trauma Foundation, AANS, CNS)*

1. Avoid hyperventilation in the first 24 hours after injury
2. Prophylactic hyperventilation ($PaCO_2 \leq 25$) is not recommended
3. Hyperventilation is recommended as a temporizing measure for lowering increased ICP
4. If hyperventilation is used, monitor O_2 delivery with jugular venous O_2 Sat (S_jO_2) or brain tissue O_2 tension ($PbrO_2$)

*These recommendations are summarized from the Guidelines for the Management of Severe Traumatic Brain Injury, 3rd Edition, 2007. BrainTrauma.org. They were a joint project of the Brain Trauma Foundation, AANS, CNS, and the AANS/CNS Joint Section on Neurotrauma and Critical Care

- PPV and PEEP can ↑ ICP because Palv is easily transmitted to vascular space in patients with normal lungs: A large ↑ in Paw, (due to ↑ $\dot{V}E$ to cause hyperventilation and ↓ ICP) may cause a paradoxical ↑ in ICP.
- PEEP < 10 cmH_2O will rarely adversely affect ICP and any effect can usually be offset by head elevation.
- Suctioning and CPT can dramatically ↑ ICP. Therefore, perform bronchial hygiene with extreme caution.

3 Strategic Pathways:

1. **Patients with Normal ICP**: Maintain normal ABG

2. **Patients with Increased ICP**:
   - Only utilize when ICP > 20 mmHg for > 5-10 min (brief increases may occur during coughing, movement, suctioning, asynchrony)
   - Elevate HOB 30° (maximizes venous outflow from head)
   - Minimize risk of Valsalva responses (suctioning)
   - Minimize cough (which increases ICP)

Hyperventilation

(controversial, no evidence to support decreased mortality)

24-48 hrs post-injury	Avoid Hyperventilation
> 48 hours post-injury	May consider mild-to-moderate hyperventilation, but avoid $PaCO_2$ < 30 mmHg[1] $PaCO_2$ 30-35 mmHg causes arteriole vasoconstriction, decreasing ICP Duration of action = 1-24 hours (brain then "resets" to new $PaCO_2$ level)
Weaning	Do NOT return to normal rapidly due to risk of rebound increase in ICP (taper over several hours)

[1] $PaCO_2$ < 30 mmHg may induce hypoxemia in brain tissue, limit oxygen delivery, and cause anaerobic metabolism/acidosis

3. <u>Neurogenic pulmonary edema</u>

Acute head injury with ↑ ICP may cause neurogenic pulmonary edema, which is clinically indistinguishable from ARDS. Treat similar to ARDS with extra caution on increasing ICP (See ARDS).

Monitoring

- Effective monitoring should be instituted to allow a rapid ↑ in ventilation and oxygenation should hypoxemia or ↑ ICP occur.
- Monitor closely for: Hypoxemia, auto-PEEP, ↑ ICP (during suctioning, CPT, and following ventilator changes), and pulmonary emboli and infections.

Weaning

Criteria for weaning:

- Normalized $PaCO_2$
- No respiratory depressant drugs in use
- Ventilatory drive intact

11 Effects and Cautions

CONTENTS

Pulmonary

Airway Obstruction 11-2
Atelectasis 11-2
Auto-PEEP (Air-Trapping) 11-3
  Measuring 11-5
  Methods to Reduce 11-6
Oxygen Toxicity 11-7
Pulmonary Vascular Resistance 11-7
Respiratory Drive (decreased) 11-7
Ventilation/Perfusion Imbalances 11-8
Work of Breathing (increased) 11-8
  Methods to Decrease 11-9
Ventilator-Associated Lung Injuries 11-10
  Injury Cascade 11-11
  Lung Protective Strategies 11-11
  Methods to Minimize Over-Distension 11-12

Arterial Blood Gases

Hypoxemia 11-12
Hypoventilation 11-13
Hyperventilation 11-13

General Considerations

Selected Effects on Body Systems 11-14
Infection 11-15
Ventilator-Associated Events 11-15

Pulmonary

Airway Obstruction

Causes	Patient	• Bronchospasm • Inadequate suctioning and/or bronchial hygiene
	Circuit	• ET tube displaced, kinked, or cuff herniation • H_2O in circuit
Signs & Symptoms	Patient	• Adventitious sounds • ↓ PaO_2 • ↑ WOB
	Machine	• ↑ PIP (Volume Ventilation) • Patient-ventilator asynchrony

Atelectasis

Causes	Patient	• Inadequate turning • Inadequate Bronchial Hygiene • ↑ Secretions/obstructions
	Machine	• High F_IO_2 (> 70%) • Low V_T • Sub-optimal PEEP
Signs & Symptoms	Patient	• ↓ BS • Crackles • ↓ PaO_2
	Machine	• ↑ PIP (VV) • ↓ V_T (PV)

Auto-PEEP (Air Trapping)

Definition	**Unintentional PEEP during Mechanical Ventilation when inspiration begins before exhalation is complete, resulting in air trapped in the lungs.** *Also known as: Breath stacking, dynamic hyperinflation, inadvertent PEEP, intrinsic PEEP, occult PEEP*	
Causes	**Patient**	↑ ***Expiratory Raw or airway collapse on exhalation:*** • Ball-valve obstruction • Bonchospasm • COPD (collapse) • Mucosal Edema • Secretions ***Active Exhalation without air-trapping*** • Increased $\dot{V}_E$ (pain, fever, ARDS)
	Machine	***Short T_E:*** • Long T_I • Slow $\dot{V}_I$ • High f • High/Inverse I:E ratio ***Mechanical expiratory Raw:*** • ET Tube • Exhalation valve, PEEP valve
Signs & Symptoms	**Patient**	• ↑ A-P Diameter (Barrel Chest) • ↑ Radiolucency on CXR • ↑ Resonance on percussion • ↑ WOB
	Machine	• Graphics (see below) • ↑ PIP in Volume Modes • ↑ P_{Plat} • ↓ Synchrony

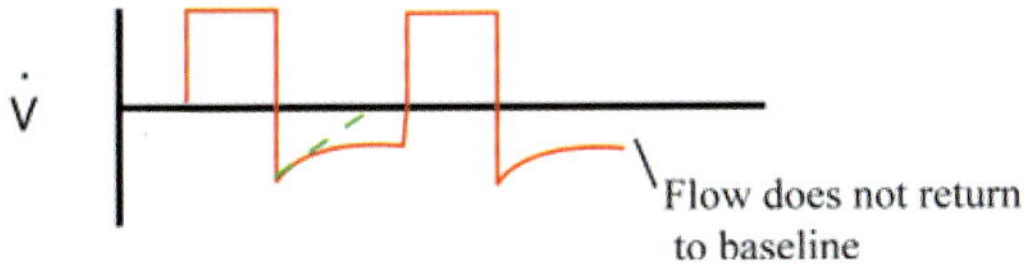

Clinical Effects	• Alveolar overdistension • Flattened hemidiaphragms • Hemodynamic compromise • Patient-Ventilator dyssynchrony • ↓ Compliance • ↓ Efficiency of pulmonary muscles • ↑ Effort to trigger ventilator • ↑ Risk of Volutrauma	
Identifying (Known)	1. *Flow / time curve:* **Expiratory flow fails to return to zero before next inspiration begins (see below)** 2. *Respirometer*: Connect a respirometer to patient's ET tube. The needle is moving when next inspiration begins.	
Identifying (Suspected)	**Patient**	• Accessory muscle use • ↓ BS, ↓ chest wall movement • Dyspnea • CXR: ↑ radiolucency, flattened hemidiaphragms • Inspiratory efforts do not trigger ventilator • Patient exhaling when next breath starts • Prolonged time constant • Patient's RR > ventilator response rate (assumes sensitivity is set properly)
	Ventilator	• ↑ PIP and P_{plat} • Transient ↓ in exhaled V_T's • High ventilator rates (AC)

Measuring Auto-PEEP

End-Expiratory Pause	• The exhalation valve is occluded for 1 – 2 sec. (some up to 4 sec) just prior to next inspiration; inspiration is delayed. • As Palv equilibrates with the proximal Paw, the level of auto-PEEP is reflected on the pressure gauge during the pause (accuracy is questionable). • Auto-PEEP = total PEEP – set PEEP • $PEEP_I = PEEP_{tot} - PEEP_E$
T-Piece Adapter (Braschi Valve)	• A T-piece adaptor with a one-way valve and cap. • The cap is removed during exhalation. • While the next mechanical breath is diverted out the uncapped hole, the pressure equilibrates between the patient's lungs and circuit. • Auto-PEEP pressure is read on a manometer proximal to the patient.
Pplat Estimate	• Measure P_{plat} during VV (P_{plat} #1) • Place on CPAP for 30 sec • Return to Volume Mode and measure P_{plat} on 1st or 2nd breath (P_{plat} # 2) • P_{plat} 1 – P_{plat} 2 = rough estimate of auto-PEEP

Clinical Note: Measuring auto-PEEP by end-expiratory pressure requires a quiet patient on controlled ventilation (i.e., no spontaneous breathing) and a circuit with no leaks.
Newer ventilators may directly measure auto-PEEP.

Effects/Cautions

Methods to Reduce Auto-PEEP

1. **Increase Expiratory Time (T_E) by:**
   - Decreasing Rate (↑ T_E)
   - Decreasing V_T (↓ T_I)
   - Decreasing Inspiratory Time
   - Increasing Flow (↓ T_I)

2. **Airflow Obstruction**
   - Administer bronchodilators (aggressively)
   - Bronchial Hygiene (lavage? therapeutic bronch?)
   - Steroid administration
   - Consider changing to larger ET Tube

3. **Decrease Minute Ventilation**
   - Treat pain
   - Treat fever

4. **Allow as much spontaneous breathing as possible:**
   - Pressure Support Ventilation (with adequate support)
   - CPAP (less common, PSV is preferred)
   - SIMV (may increase dyssynchrony so assess closely)

5. **Apply PEEP/CPAP (up to 80 % of auto-PEEP)**
   Carefully ↑ applied PEEP in increments of 1 cmH_2O until the patient's rate and the ventilator rate are equal. (Applied PEEP > auto-PEEP may lead to further hyperinflation and complications).

6. **Lower resistance exhalation valve (if available)**

Clinical Note: Permissive hypercapnia is sometimes recommended when auto-PEEP cannot be reduced due to high $\dot{V}_E$ demand and/or severe airway obstruction.

Oxygen Toxicity

Causes	$F_IO_2 > 0.6$ for > 48 hrs
Signs & Symptoms	• ↓ PaO_2 • ↑ $PA\text{-}aO_2$ • ↓ Compliance • ↑WOB • ↑ V/Q mismatch

Pulmonary Vascular Resistance (PVR)

PVR changes are complex and dependent on the patient's pathophysiology, and the level and mode of MV – which is beyond the scope of this book.

Respiratory Drive Decreased

Causes	• Overventilation • CO_2 narcosis • Sedation • Overdose
Signs & Symptoms	• Absence of breathing (Apnea)* • ↓ $PaCO_2$ (rate too high on ventilator) • Patient riding rate on ventilator (Patient RR = Ventilator *f*) • ↑ $PaCO_2$ • ↓ PaO_2

* This may particularly be noted when switching suddenly to a spontaneous mode (PSV) from A/C with a high ventilator rate. The patient has no drive to breathe until their CO_2 has had a chance to rise adequately. This, at times, is mistaken for weaning failure.

Effects/Cautions

Ventilation/Perfusion (V/Q) Imbalances

Causes	• The relationship of ventilation (flow of air) and perfusion (flow of blood) affects gas exchange efficiency
	• V/Q imbalances are complex and dependent on a patient's pathophysiology and the level/ mode of ventilation. Common causes include:
	  • Atelectasis
	  • Consolidation (e.g. Pneumonia)
	  • Pulmonary Edema
	  • ARDS
	  • Reduced Hemoglobin

Signs & Symptoms	• Refractory Hypoxemia • Hypercapnia • Confusion/Somnolence

Work of Breathing (WOB)

Causes	**Patient**	• ↓ C_L (various) • High inspiratory flow demand (various) • ↑ Raw (various)
	Circuit	• Inadequate $\dot{V}_I$ • Insensitive trigger • Inadequate demand valve (SIMV) • High resistance circuits, ET tubes, humidifiers, PEEP, and/or exhalation valves.
Signs & Symptoms	**Patient**	• Accessory muscle use • ↑ Spontaneous rate • Restlessness / anxiety • Nasal Flaring • Diaphoresis • Retractions
	Machine	• Asynchrony • ↑ PIP

Effects/Cautions

Strategies to Reduce WOB

1. **Consider Patient-ventilator synchronization:**
   - $\dot{V}_I$ to match patient demand (usually 60 – 100 L/min)
   - Proper machine sensitivity (most sensitive possible without auto-triggering)
   - Proper $\dot{V}_I$ pattern
   - Proper mode (may need to trial several)

2. **Decrease Raw:**
   - Larger ET tube
   - Keep ET tube free of secretions and kinks
   - Use of bronchodilators

3. **Increase Compliance:**
   - Diuretics to reduce edema in lung parenchyma
   - Pleural drainage to eliminate pleural fluid or air
   - Semi-Fowler position (or greater)

4. **Decrease Minute Ventilation Requirement:**

   Reduce or eliminate:
   - agitation
   - anxiety
   - fever
   - pain
   - seizures

5. **Consider PSV and/or PEEP:**

   To reduce any WOB not corrected by above:
   - Perform Optimal PEEP Maneuver (see Optimal PEEP)
   - Consider addition of Pressure Support to spontaneous breaths

Ventilator Associated Lung Injury (VALI)
Ventilator Induced Lung Injury (VILI)

Definition and Factors		**VILI** = acute lung injury caused by ventilator **VALI** = injury not proven to be caused by vent. ***Primary factors:*** **1. Mechanical** • Barotrauma (Atelectrauma, Volutrauma) • Length of ventilation • Patient positioning **2. Biological** • Biotrauma (cytokine release due to epithelial injury from baro/volutrauma) • Hyperoxia (fibrotic, absorption atelectasis) **3. Pathological** (disease process)
Cause 1: Over-distension *High ventilating pressures can produce high distending volumes, leading to alveolar over-distension in areas of high lung compliance. See Damage Cascade on next page.*		
Specific Causes	**Patient**	• ARDS (late stage) • ↑ C_L (bullous or necrotizing lung disease, emphysema) • Rt mainstem intubation
	Machine	• High airway pressures [high V_T, PIP, Palv (PPlat) PEEP] *
Signs & Symptoms	**Patient**	• Arrhythmias • ↓ BP • ↓ BS • ↑ Chest expansion (affected side) • ↓ PaO_2 • ↑ WOB
	Machine	↑ PIP (Volume modes) ↑ PPlat
Cause 2: De-recruitment Injury *Alveolar collapse at end-expiration leads to repeated opening and closing of alveoli, resulting in shear force injury (atelectrauma)*		

Damage begins a cascade of:

Trauma → Air Leak → ↑Vascular Permeability → Fluid/Protein shifts across A-C Membrane → High Permeability Pulmonary Edema → Surfactant Disturbance → Alveolar Instability → ↓ CL → V/Q Mismatch → Shunting → ↓ Gas Exchange → Activated immunological response → Release of Inflammatory Mediators (Cytokines) → Neutrophil Aggregation → Fibrin Deposits → Fibrotic Changes → Widened Air/Blood Interface → ↓ FRC → Systemic Inflammatory Response (SIRS) → ↑ Morbidity and Mortality

Lung Protective Strategies

Reduce Positive Pressure Ventilation	• Low V_T (6-8 cc/kg IBW) (prevent overdistension) • Low PIP (< 30 cmH_2O) (prevent overdistension) • Permissive hypoxemia (minimize mechanical effects of PPV) • Permissive hypercapnia (minimize mechanical effects of PPV) • Rapid weaning (minimize time of PPV)
Open Lung Approach	• Adequate PEEP (minimize shearing, prevent derecruitment, maximize ventilation) • Lung recruitment (overcome the closing pressure and minimize threshold opening pressure of collapsed alveoli): • Sustained inflation • PEEP manipulation • Prone positioning (passive maintenance of lung recruitment)
Alternative Strategies	• APRV • HFOV • NPPV • NAVA • Surfactant replacement therapy • ECMO • Anti-cytokine therapies

Methods for Minimizing Over-Distension

- Use low V_T strategy
- ↓ V_T as ↑ PEEP
- Keep P_{plat} < 30 cmH_2O
- Avoid Right Mainstem Intubation
- Monitor use of PEEP carefully (ensure optimal)
- Minimize/correct auto-PEEP
- Consider permissive hypercapnia

Arterial Blood Gases

Hypoxemia

Causes	**Patient**	• Various: See Oakes' ABG Pocket Guide for a detailed explanation
	Machine	• Low FiO_2 • Vent/Circuit malfunction • O_2 analyzer calibration problem
Signs & Symptoms	**Patient**	• ↓ PaO_2 • ↑ WOB ***compensatory responses to hypoxemia:*** • ↑ HR • ↑ RR, if able

Hypoventilaton

Causes	**Patient**	↑ $\dot{V}_E$ demand
	Machine	↓ $\dot{V}_E$ delivered
Signs & Symptoms	**Patient**	↑ $PaCO_2$, ↓ pH ↑ WOB

Hypoventilation can lead to:

Potential hypoxemia (in absence of supplemental O_2):

- Rt shift of O_2-Hgb dissociation curve (↓ Hgb binding of O_2)
- ↑ $PaCO_2$ leads to ↓ PaO_2

Hyperkalemia (cardiac dysrhythmias)

↑ ICP in patients with cerebral disorders

> **Clinical Notes: Hypercapnia with moderate acidosis is not as harmful as high level ventilation to maintain normocapnia. Rapid ↑ $PaCO_2$ and ↓ pH can lead to coma.**

Hyperventilation

Causes	**Patient**	↓ $\dot{V}_E$ demand Hypoxia
	Machine	↑ $\dot{V}_E$ delivered
Signs & Symptoms	**Patient**	↓ $PaCO_2$, ↑ pH

Hyperventilation can lead to:

Lung Injury, ↓ CO

Hypokalemia (cardiac dysrrhythmias)

Lt shift of O_2-Hgb dissociation curve (↑ Hgb binding resulting in less O_2 available at tissue level)

> **Clinical Notes: Prolonged, severe hypocapnia can lead to tetany and ↓ cerebral perfusion. Normocapnia in chronic CO_2 retainers is indicative of relative hyperventilation.**

Selected Effects of Positive Pressure Ventilation on Body Systems*

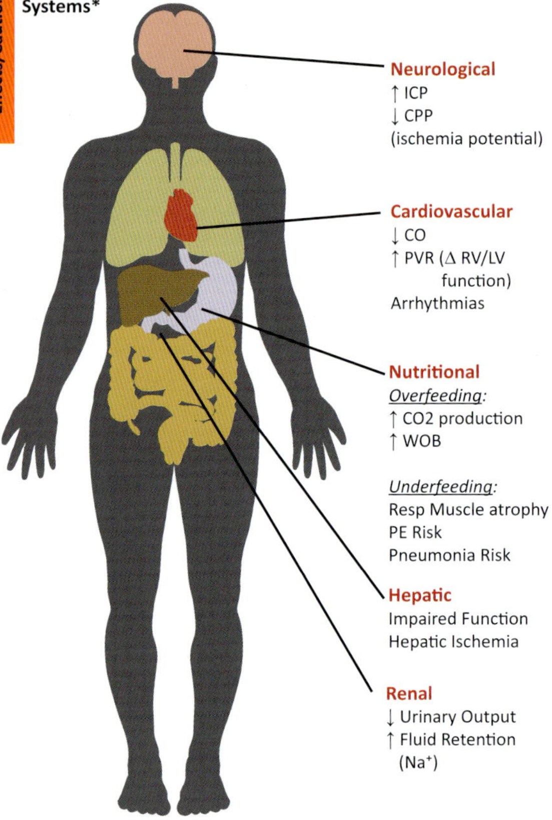

****This is intended to be a summary. For more complete information see RespiratoryUpdate.com or Oakes' Critical Care Pocket Guide.***

Infection

Causes	**Patient**	• ↓ resistance • Aspiration	
	Machine	• Unsterile technique • ET Tube microaspiration/cuff leak	
Signs & Symptoms	**Patient**	• Cough • Diaphoresis • Fever • ↑ HR • ↑ WBC	• possible CXR Infiltrates • Sputum production (amount, color, consistency)

Ventilator Associated Events (VAE)

(formerly: Ventilator Associated Pneumonia [VAP])

VAE Prevention

1. Avoid Intubation (consider NPPV)
2. When Intubated:

A. Ventilator Bundle	1. HOB 30° - 45° 2. Daily sedation vacation 3. Peptic Ulcer Disease (PUD) prophylaxis 4. Deep Venous Thrombosis (DVT) prophylaxis 5. Daily oral care with chlorhexidine
B. Prevent bacterial colonization of upper airway	• Avoid unnecessary antibiotic use • Chlorhexidine oral rinse in high-risk patients • Isolation precautions (patients infected with high-risk pathogens) • Oral hygiene and decontamination • Routine hand washing (with alcohol rubs) and glove
C. Prevent aspiration of contaminated secretions into the lower airways	• Avoid unnecessary use of sedation • Avoid gastric overdistention • Discontinue NG/ET tubes ASAP • Drainage of ventilator circuit condensate • ET tube cuff pressure > 20 cmH_2O • Limit saline instillation with suctioning • Subglottic drainage

D. Other	• Avoid paralytics when possible • Change ventilator circuit only when visibly soiled or non-functioning • Immunize healthcare workers for influenza • Maintain patient's immune defenses and nutritional status • Prefer noninvasive ventilation • Use HME or heated wire circuit instead of active humidifier. • Use closed (in-line) suction catheters

Notes Page

Make It Your Own

Notes Page

12 Discontinuation / Weaning

CONTENTS

Definitions 12-2

Discontinuation Assessment

Primary Pathology 12-3
Vital Signs 12-3
Respiratory Assessment 12-4
  Predictive indices 12-4
  Acid-Base Balance 12-6
  Airway 12-6
  Chest X-Ray 12-7
  Ventilatory Muscles 12-7
  Ventilatory Drive and Demand 12-7
Cardiovascular Assessment 12-8
Electrolyte Assessment 12-8
Metabolic Assessment 12-8
Neurologic Assessment 12-9
Nutritional Assessment 12-9
Pharmacological Assessment 12-9
Psychological Assessment 12-10
Renal Assessment 12-11
Miscellaneous Factors 12-11
Procedural Factors 12-11

Discontinuation Methods

Abrupt Discontinuation 12-12
Gradual Weaning 12-12

Other Considerations

ACCP Discontinuation/Weaning 12-15
Monitoring of Success or Failure 12-21
  RSBI 12-22
Weaning 12-23
Extubation
  Assessment 12-24
  Procedure 12-25
Post-Extubation Care 12-26

Definitions

Discontinuation	The permanent removal from the ventilator
Liberation	The ability to breathe without the assistance of the ventilator
Weaning*	The gradual reduction of ventilator support and its replacement with spontaneous ventilation
Progressive withdrawal	Refers to the gradual (weaning) approach of discontinuation
Readiness Testing	The initial period of minimal ventilatory support for evaluation of abrupt discontinuation
Spontaneous Breathing Trial (SBT)	A period of up to 30 - 120 minutes in which a patient breathes with little or no help from the ventilator. A successful trial lasts 30-120 minutes, and implies no further need for mechanical ventilation.
Ventilatory Demand	≈ CO_2 production/retention
Ventilatory capacity	≈ Drive to breath (CNS) and muscles ability to breathe (strength and endurance)
Ability to wean	Ventilatory capacity > ventilatory demand
Inability to wean	Ventilatory capacity < ventilatory demand
Discontinuation failure	The need to re-institute ventilatory support
Ventilator-dependent	Patients who need MV beyond 24 hours or those who have failed discontinuation attempts.
Extubation	The removal of the artificial airway

Discontinuation Assessment

There are many tools for assessing readiness to wean/extubate/discontinue ventilator support. None of these alone will predict success in all cases. Clinical judgment, including a professional weighing of the risks and benefits, is important.

Intubated Patients: Discontinuing means extubating, with the major risk being the need to reintubate (which increases the risk of aspiration, trauma, or a major event like a code). This requires clinicians to be relatively conservative in making a decision to extubate.

Tracheostomy Patients: Discontinuing means disconnecting the ventilator, but the artificial airway remains. The risks are less here, suggesting clinicians can be more aggressive in attempting to liberate from the ventilator.

Note: Each factor should be optimized before attempting the discontinuation process. Although every problem need not be resolved before discontinuation, major problems should be corrected and the other areas need to be assessed as to their cumulative effect on inhibiting the discontinuation process.

Resolution of the acute phase of the cause (disease) is the most important indicator of readiness for discontinuation.

Items in orange throughout the following sections should be considered as the minimum required assessment. Many other assessment options listed should be used as clinically appropriate.

Vital Signs

Parameter	RR	HR	BP	Temp
Desired Value	≤ 30 breaths/min	≤ 140 bpm	stable with no/minimal pressors	Normal (< 38° C)

Respiratory Assessment

Below, plus see Chapter 5 for Patient - Ventilator Assessment and Trouble-Shooting.

Predictive Indices (see chapter 7 for Equations)

- *Unless otherwise indicated these indices assume minimal ventilator support with spontaneous effort*
- *Items in orange are most common indices used clinically. The others are listed for reference*

Oxygenation

Parameter	Desired/Threshold Value
$PaO_2 \le 0.4\text{-}0.5\ FiO_2$	> 60 mmHg
SaO_2 on FiO_2 up to 0.4	> 90%
PaO_2/FiO_2 ratio	> 200
PaO_2/PAO_2	> 0.35
$P(A\text{-}a)O_2$	< 350 mmHg on FiO_2 = 1.0
Q_S/Q_T (shunt %)	< 0.2 (20%)
Hgb	> 8-10 g/dL
Low PEEP	< 8 cmH_2O

Ventilation

Parameter	Desired/Threshold Value
$PaCO_2$	< 50 mmHg
$\dot{V}_E$ (spont.)	< 10 to 15 L/min
V_D/V_T	< 0.6
V_T (Spontaneous)	> 5 cc/kg IBW
Respiratory rate (spont.)	< 35/min or > 6-10/min
Respiratory pattern	Regular

Mechanics

Parameter	Desired/Threshold Value
P_{IMAX} (MIF, MIP, NIF)	more negative than - 20 to - 30 cmH_2O
VC	> 10 - 15 mL/kg
MVV	≥ 2 x spontaneous $\dot{V}_E$ (resting) or > 20 L/min
C_{dyn}	≥ 22 mL/cmH_2O
C_{stat}	≥ 33 mL/cmH_2O
$P_{0.1}$	≤ 6 cmH_2O

Integrated Indices

Parameter	Desired/Threshold Value
RSBI (f/V_T)*	< 105 breaths/min/L
SWI (Simplified Weaning Index)	< 9/min
CROP index	> 13 mL/breaths/min
$P_{0.1}/P_{IMAX}$	< 0.9

*Some clinicians use a lower RSBI than 105 to determine readiness

Acid-Base Balance / Metabolic Status

Remember, pH is more important than $PaCO_2$ / HCO_3 in general. Acid-Base balance should be achieved before proceeding with wean.

Imbalance	Causes	Effects
Respiratory Acidosis	Hypoventilation	↑ ventilatory demand
Respiratory Alkalosis	Hyperventilation	↓ ventilatory drive ↑ Hgb affinity for O_2
Metabolic Acidosis	Lactic acidosis Ketoacidosis	↑ ventilatory demand Confusion Pulmonary edema Arrhythmias (severe)
Metabolic Alkalosis	↓ K^+, CL^- Nasogastric tube Vomiting	↓ ventilatory drive ↑ Hgb affinity for O_2

Discontinuation

Airway

Assess for:	Goal
Obstruction	Verify via auscultation, CXR, etc. that there is no acute obstruction (anatomic, broncho-spasm, etc.)
Gag Reflex	This can often be noted during routine oral care. If not, very gently insert a small FR suction catheter toward the back of the tongue
Airway Patency	Consider cuff leak test if patency is questionable (many consider ANY leak acceptable, but issues such as too large of an ET Tube should also be considered)
Secretions	Patients should be able to clear secretions on their own if being extubated. Note cough (MIP) ability, amount of secretions, consistency of secretions

Chest X-ray

Chest X-ray (CXR) should be systematically reviewed, including comparing several from different dates, when available. Any acute processes (that contributed to failure) should be resolved or resolving.

Ventilatory Muscles/Strength

Bedside Assessment: Ask patient to hold their head up off the pillow for about 10 seconds. This indicates adequate strength and confirms the ability to follow instruction

Major causes of concern with strength include patient being deconditioned from prolonged ventilator support. This can best be addressed proactively by using early mobility strategies, aggressive weaning, etc. Other concerns include decreased capacity (drugs, malnutrition, sleep deprivation, etc.) and increased load (small ET Tube, ↓ compliance, chestwall restrictions such as obesity)

Ventilatory Drive and Demand

Factors that ↑ Ventilatory Drive	Factors that ↓ Ventilatory Drive
• Acidosis • Agitation • Anxiety • Closed head injury • Drugs (stimulants) • Dyspnea • Fear • Hypoxia • Pain	• Alkalosis • CNS injury or disease • Drugs (depressants) • Electrolyte imbalance • Fatigue • ↓ metabolism • Sedation

Factors that increase Ventilatory Demand:

- ↑ Ventilatory drive (see above)
- ↑ $\dot{V}CO_2$ (See Metabolic Assessment)
- ↑ V_D: Anatomical, mechanical

Discontinuation

Discontinuation

Cardiovascular Assessment

Below, plus see also chapter 5: *Assessment and Troubleshooting*

Parameter	Desired/Threshold Value
Stable BP	Stable with minimal pressor/inotropic support
Fluid Imbalance	If significantly +, consider diuresing pt prior to extubation
Anemia	Check Hgb and Hct
Hemo Stability	Verify adequate CO, no shock, adeq. LV function, contractility, stable EKG

Electrolyte Assessment

Parameter	Normal Range	Significance
Phosphate (PO_4)	1.4 - 2.7 mg/dL	Decreases in these values may indicate a diminished ventilatory drive
Potassium (K^+)	3.5 - 5.0 mEq/L	
Magnesium (Mg^+)	1.3 - 2.5 mEq/L	

Metabolism

↑ Metabolism (↑ $\dot{V}co_2$)	↓ Metabolism (↓ $\dot{V}co_2$)
• Agitation • Excessive caloric intake (See Nutritional Assessment) • Fever • Seizures • Sepsis • Shivering • Tremors • ↑ WOB	• Malnutrition • Starvation (↓ ventilatory drive and muscles)

Neurologic Assessment

In Neuro Injury/Disease, Use Caution if:

- ICP > 20 mmHg
- CPP < 60 mmHg
- Seizures

Also consider CNS Drive (see Ventilatory Drive), Mental Status (see Psychological Assessment), and Musculature (see Ventilatory Muscles)

Discontinuation

Nutritional Assessment

Undernourished	Overnourished
• Resp Muscle atrophy • PE Risk • Pneumonia/Infection Risk	• ↑ CO_2 production • ↑ WOB • ↑ $\dot{V}E$ requirement (with high carb load)

Appropriate caloric intake

- Appropriate nutrition-caloric intake: 1.5 - 2 x REE (resting energy expenditure)
- Appropriate protein intake: 1 - 1.5 gm/kg/day

Pharmacological Assessment

Drug Type	Potential Effects
• Hypnotics • **Sedatives** • Narcotics • Tranquilizers	↓ Ventilatory drive and/or mental response
• Stimulants	↑ Ventilatory drive
• Aminoglycosides (potentiates NMBAs) • Corticosteroids • Muscle Relaxants • **Neuromuscular blockers (NMBA)**	↓ Ventilatory muscle function

Psychological Assessment

There are many psychological factors to consider, some predictable and others not. This list is not exhaustive, but looks at some of the most common considerations:

Factor	Considerations
Anxiety/Fear	• Communicate clearly with patient • Have familiar faces at bedside • Consider anti-anxiety drugs
Combativeness	• Ensure no drug/alcohol abuse history • Consider change in sedation (such as to Precedex) • Accelerate extubation if clinically acceptable (combativeness may be related to fear/claustrophobia)
Delirium	• Consider pharmacological intervention
Pain	• Ask patient about pain, if able or • Manage pain by watching for patient cues (grimacing, etc.) and vitals
Psychological Dependence on Ventilator	• Use slow wean strategy - small steps
Sleep Deprivation	• Ensure Pt-Vent Synchrony • Create environment that mimics day/night (minimize as many pt care interactions as possible at night, keep noise to a minimum at night) • Consider sleep aids (eye mask, earplugs, white noise)
Withdrawal (drugs, alcohol)	• Consider with team: may require pharmacologic treatment • Patient may need to remain intubated until acute withdrawal symptoms have passed

Renal Assessment

Renal Factors	Comments
Acid-base abnormalities	Affects drive and load
Fluid imbalance / I & O / Renal Insufficiency	Overload impairs pulmonary gas exchange and leads to pulmonary edema (Adequate output > 1000 mL/day and equal to intake)
Electrolyte imbalance	Causes ventilatory muscle weakness

Miscellaneous Factors

- Exercise tolerance
- Gastrointestinal (stress-related hemorrhage, inability to tolerate enteral nutrition, bowel obstruction, ascites)
- Hyperglycemia
- Infection/sepsis (↑ $\dot{V}CO_2$ +$\dot{V}O_2$)
- Impending surgical procedures requiring general anesthetics
- Malpositioning

Procedural factors

- *Improper weaning procedures*:
  Time of day (avoid evenings, nights, and shift change)
  Inadequate staffing
  Interruptions and disruptions
- *Improper technical factors*:
  Inappropriate support level
  Inappropriate sensitivity level
  Inappropriate PEEP level

Discontinuation Methods*

Method	Description	Technique/Procedure	Comments
Abrupt Discontinuation			
Spontaneous Breathing Trial (SBT) ***Readiness Testing***	A period of 30 - 120 minutes in which patients breathe with little or no help from the ventilator.	**Off Ventilator:** T-piece with or without low level CPAP (e.g., 5cmH_2O). Use adequate continuous flow. **On Ventilator:** 1) Spontaneous breathing through a flow-triggering ventilator with or without low level CPAP (e.g., 5cmH_2O) 2) Spontaneous breathing with low level PSV. Use minimal PS to offset ET tube resistance.	Most recommended method for the majority of patients. If the patient is not extubated, rest at night on non-fatiguing ventilatory support.
Gradual Weaning			
1) PSV	Reducing the PS level as the patient's respiratory muscles strengthen	Begin with a PS level at which the respiratory rate and V_T are close to full (PS_{MAX}) or partial ventilatory support (maintain minute volume). Gradually ↓ the PS level as tolerated. The most appropriate level is that just high enough to prevent activation of accessory muscles. Continue to a minimal level (~5-10 cmH_2O) to overcome resistance of the artificial airway and ventilator circuit. Discontinue when the patient can maintain this minimal level.	Most preferred method of gradual weaning. It works best for short-term weaning (< 72 hours). If it is used in long-term weaning, increase support at night to near maximum to allow patient to rest and sleep.

Method	Description	Technique/Procedure	Comments
2) SIMV	Volume or pressure machine breaths synchronized with the patient's spontaneous breaths.	Decrease the mandatory (machine) breaths as tolerated, requiring the patient to assume more of the responsibility for the minute volume. Discontinue when the patient can maintain for 1-2 hours at a rate of 4 breaths/minute.	Related to the poorest weaning outcomes due to the fatiguing load of the mandatory breaths. Patient/ventilator asynchrony may occur at low rates. Works best for short-term weaning. If used for long-term weaning, increase support at night to near maximum to allow the patient to rest and sleep. PS at low levels (5-10 cmH_2O) is commonly added to help overcome resistance of the ET tube (or automatic tube compensation, if available)

Method	Description	Technique/Procedure	Comments
3) SBT On or off the ventilator (*T-Piece*)	Gradually increasing period of time (length of time and number of times/ day) off ventilatory support.	*Same as SBT above*: Start with 5 minutes of spontaneous breathing Work up to 20-30 minutes with appropriate rest intervals on the ventilator. Gradually increase the amount of time of spontaneous breathing plus decrease the intervals of rest. When using the ventilator, PS and/or CPAP can be added.	Patients should not be required to breathe through a ET tube for > 30-60 minutes due to ↑ WOB. Any patient who can last 30 minutes is probably ready to be discontinued and possibly extubated. (See Abrupt)
4) NPPV (Noninvasive Positive Pressure Ventilation)	The method used when a patient no longer requires an artificial airway, but does need ventilatory support.	As a patient is extubated, NPPV may be needed to ventilate the patient noninvasively to prevent reintubation. A mask covers the nose or full face in which positive pressure is delivered.	Prevents the complications of invasive ventilation. See Chapter 9.

* **Clinical Notes**: Any combination of the above gradual weaning methods may also be used.

Automated weaning approaches (MMV, VS, VAPS, etc) may be an option. There is currently no evidence that these modes improve weaning outcomes.

The method chosen should be based on careful patient assessment, clinical experience, and a sound protocol, which should be individualized for that particular patient. See Page 13-13.

ACCP Discontinuation/Weaning Guidelines

General Guidelines (Regardless of method)

Provide explanation and encouragement to the patient.

Preferably done during the day to allow the patient to rest at night; avoid weaning during shift change

Do not fatigue the patient's ventilatory muscles (i.e., do not "wean to exhaustion"). Monitor clinical signs closely.

Clinical Recommendations of ACCP 2001 †

Start discontinuation or weaning of MV soon after initiation, by developing a protocol that assesses readiness.

Regardless of the technique used, a non-physician, healthcare professional-driven protocol significantly expedites safe weaning.

For cardiac surgery, a rapid protocol allows early extubation.

The role for computerized protocols has not been established.

No weaning parameters (predictors) have been proven. However, some do have better predictive power than others, such as RSBI (f / V_T), CROP, and PaO_2/F_IO_2.

SBT and PSV techniques are superior to IMV.

Early identification of readiness (followed by extubation or extubation with NPPV) is beneficial and prevents MV complications related to unnecessary delays.

† Adapted from ACCP/AARC/SCCM Evidence-Based Guidelines for Weaning and Discontinuing Ventilatory Support, ***Chest***, Vol. 120, # 6, supplement, 2001.

*Clinical Recommendations of ACCP 1993**

Do not begin weaning until evidence of significant improvement in the initial precipitating illness.

Routinely evaluate pt's ability to sustain spontaneous ventilation

Stop/modify weaning process if insufficiency and/or distress appear, persist, or worsen. Avoid ↑ WOB imposed by breathing circuits, demand valves, and small ET tubes.

SIMV weaning should be guided by pH, $PaCO_2$, total RR, HR, and signs of distress.

Know the signs of ↑ ventilatory insufficiency and patient distress:

↑ Tachypnea (> 30 - 35 breaths/min)	↑ HR	↓ pH (< 7.25 –7.30) and
	Pain	↑ $PaCO_2$
Diaphoresis		Unrelieved agitation

* Adapted from ACCP Consensus Conference: Mechanical Ventilation, ***Respiratory Care***, Vol. 38, #12, 1993.

ACCP/AARC/SCCM Evidenced-Based Guidelines for Weaning and Discontinuation of Ventilatory Support (1)(2)

Patients requiring MV > 24 hrs: Search for causes of ventilator dependence

↓

Begin to reverse causes
(See pg 13-2 for Discontinuation Assessment)

↓

Is the patient ready for formal assessment for discontinuation?

1. Evidence of some reversal of the underlying cause
2. Adequate oxygenation (exceptions can be made for chronic hypoxemic patients)
   a. $PaO_2/FiO_2 > 150\text{-}200$
   b. Requiring PEEP $\leq$ 5-8cmH_2O
   c. $FiO_2 \leq 0.4\text{-}0.5$ and pH ≥ 7.25
3. Hemodynamic stability
   a. No significant hypotension/on no or low dose vasopressors
   b. No active ischemia
4. Capability to initiate an inspiratory effort

NO → **Continue with current settings**

YES ↓

Place patient on an initial brief period (3-5 minutes) of spontaneous breathing

↓

Perform a formal discontinuation assessment during spontaneous breathing

Did the patient tolerate the initial brief period of spontaneous breathing? (3-5 minutes)

I. Objective measurements indicating tolerance/success
- 1. Acceptable gas exchange
  - a. Oxygenation
    - i. $SpO_2 \geq$ 85-90%
    - ii. $PaO_2 \geq$ 50-60 mmHg
  - b. Ventilation
    - i. Increases in $PaCO_2 \leq$10 m Hg
    - ii. pH $\geq$ 7.32
- 2. Hemodynamic stability
  - a. HR < 120-140 beats/min or < 20% change
  - b. Systolic BP < 180-200 and > 90 mmHg, BP not changed > 20% and no pressors required
- 3. Stable ventilatory pattern
  - a. RR< 30-35 breaths/min and change < 50%

II. Subjective clinical assessments indicating intolerance/failure
- 1. Change in mental status (e.g., somnolence, coma, agitation, anxiety)
- 2. Onset or worsening of discomfort
- 3. Diaphoresis
- 4. Signs of increased WOB
  - a. Use of accessory muscles
  - b. Thoracoabdominal paradox

YES ↓ NO ↓

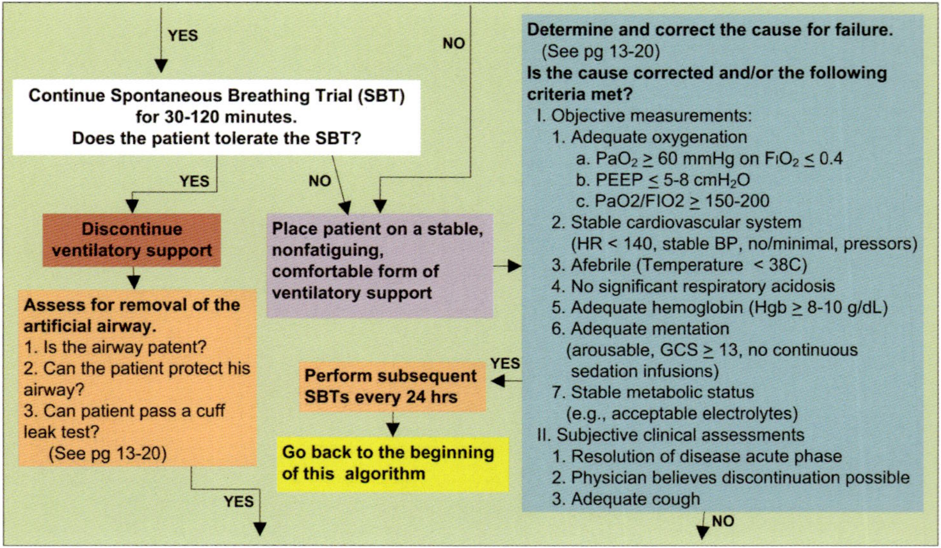
YES
NO
Continue Spontaneous Breathing Trial (SBT) for 30-120 minutes.
Does the patient tolerate the SBT?
YES
NO
Discontinue ventilatory support
Place patient on a stable, nonfatiguing, comfortable form of ventilatory support
Assess for removal of the artificial airway.
1. Is the airway patent?
2. Can the patient protect his airway?
3. Can patient pass a cuff leak test?
(See pg 13-20)
YES
Determine and correct the cause for failure.
(See pg 13-20)
Is the cause corrected and/or the following criteria met?
I. Objective measurements:
1. Adequate oxygenation
a. $PaO_2 \geq 60$ mmHg on $FiO_2 \leq 0.4$
b. PEEP $\leq$ 5-8 cmH_2O
c. PaO2/FIO2 $\geq$ 150-200
2. Stable cardiovascular system
(HR < 140, stable BP, no/minimal, pressors)
3. Afebrile (Temperature < 38C)
4. No significant respiratory acidosis
5. Adequate hemoglobin (Hgb $\geq$ 8-10 g/dL)
6. Adequate mentation
(arousable, GCS $\geq$ 13, no continuous sedation infusions)
7. Stable metabolic status
(e.g., acceptable electrolytes)
II. Subjective clinical assessments
1. Resolution of disease acute phase
2. Physician believes discontinuation possible
3. Adequate cough
YES
NO
Perform subsequent SBTs every 24 hrs
Go back to the beginning of this algorithm

In post surgical patients, anesthesia/ sedation strategies and ventilator management should aim for early extubation.

Extubate
(See pg 13-19)

Gradual discontinuation methods may be attempted. Weaning to approximately half-support as the causes of failure are gradually corrected.

Tracheotomy should be considered when it becomes apparent the the patient will require prolonged ventilatory assistance.
Tracheotomy should then be performed when the patient appears likely to gain one or more of the benefits of this procedure:

Early tracheotomy is considered in :

1. Those requiring high levels of sedation to tolerate translaryngeal tubes
2. Those with marginal respiratory mechanics (often manifested as tachypnea) in which a tracheostomy tube, having lower resistance, might reduce the risk of muscle overload
3. Those who may derive psychological benefit from the ability to:
   a. Eat orally
   b. Communicate by articulated speech
   c. Experience enhanced mobility
4. Those in whom enhanced mobility may assist physical therapy efforts

Weaning strategy in the prolonged mechanical ventilated patient should:
Be slow paced, then at half-support, switch to gradual lengthening self-breathing trials

Go back to the beginning of this algorithm

Critical care practitioners should familiarize themselves with facilities in their communities or units in their hospital that specialize and have success in managing patients who require prolonged dependence on mechanical ventilation.

Unless the disease is irreversible, a patient requiring prolonged ventilatory support for respiratory failure should not be considered permanently ventilator-dependant until 3 months of weaning attempts have failed.

When medically stable for transfer, patients who have failed ventilator discontinuation attempts in the ICU should be transferred to those facilities that have demonstrated success and safety in accomplishing ventilator discontinuation.

(1) Adapted from the ACCP/AARC/SCCM Evidence-Based Guidelines for Weaning and Discontinuing Ventilatory Support (2001)
From: *Chest* 2001;120(6)375S-395S)

(2) Protocols designed for non-physician health care professionals should be developed and implemented by ICUs:
a. Weaning/discontinuation; b. Optimizing of sedation

See AARC Clinical Practice Guidelines: ACCP MV Weaning Protocols (www.RCJournal.com/cpgs/index.cfm)

Clinical Indicators of Discontinuation/Weaning Failure

Monitor	Signs of Failure
Respiratory	
RR	> 30 - 35 breaths/min or < 10 breaths/min or > 50% change
V_T	< 5 cc/kg (< 250cc in adults)
↑ WOB	↑ Accessory muscle use Paradoxical Breathing
RSBI	> 105 breaths/min/L
ABGs/Oxygenation	
PaO_2	< 50-60 mmHg
SaO_2	< 85-90%
$PaCO_2$	↑ > 10 mmHg from baseline or > 55 mmHg (except in CO_2 retainers)
pH	↓ > 0.10 from baseline or < 7.30
Cardiovascular	
HR	Change by 20% or < 60/min or > 120 - 140/min
BP	Change > 20% systolic or 10% diastolic or < 90 mmHg or > 180 mmHg systolic > 90 mmHg diastolic
EKG	Significant arrhythmias, angina, ↑ PAWP
Other	
Δ in Mental Status	Agitation, anxiety, coma, somnolence
Diaphoresis	Present
Discomfort	Increased or pain or dyspnea

RSBI Procedure *

1. Remove the patient from ventilatory support.
2. Allow patient's spontaneous breathing pattern to stabilize.
3. Measure expired $\dot{V}_E$ and RR for one minute with respirometer (May stay on ventilator using ventilator rate of 0 and pressure support level of 0).
4. Divide $\dot{V}_E$ by frequency f to obtain average V_T.
5. Divide f by V_T to obtain RSBI (f / V_T)
   (Shortcut calculation: $f / V_T = f^2 / \dot{V}_E$)

Note that some clinicians perform RSBI with patients on minimal support settings (such as PSV 10/5).

RSBI example:	RSBI shortcut calculation example:
$\dot{V}_E$ = 10 L f = 20 breaths/min $\dot{V}_E$ / f = 10 L/20 breaths/min = 0.5L f / V_T = 20 breaths/min/0.5L = 40 breaths/min/L	$\dot{V}_E$ = 10 L f = 20 f^2 / $\dot{V}_E$ = 20 x 20 = 400/10 = 40 breaths/min/L

* Adapted from Ely EW, Baker AM, Dunagan DP, et al: Effect on the duration of mechanical ventilation of identifying patients capable of breathing spontaneously. ***N Engl J Med***, vol. 335, pp. 1864-9, 1996

Common Causes for Discontinuation Failure

Reasons for failure are the same reasons for not beginning the discontinuation process (See Discontinuation Assessment and Predictive Indices in this Chapter).

Weaning (Gradual Reduction of Ventilatory Support)

Advantages Over Abrupt Discontinuation for Some Patients

- May be tolerated better in patients who have been ventilated for long periods (> 1 week).
- Fewer risks of CV instability in patients with impaired CV system.
- Gradually increasing muscle loads in relation to the patient's ventilatory muscle recovery.

Optimal Criteria for Ventilatory Support Weaning

- Proper muscle loading (↓ ventilatory support must not lead to fatigue).
- Maximal patient-ventilator synchrony is essential.
- Frequent assessments and readjustments.

Extubation Assessment

Assessment for Removal of the Artificial Airway

- Check for airway patency
- Perform Cuff Leak Test (see below)
  If test is negative consider steroids for 24-hours before extubating*
- Assess ability to protect lower airway (Gag reflex, adequate cough)

Discontinuation

* The value of a negative cuff leak test is much debated. Note that other factors may affect a negative result, such as too large of a ET Tube.

Cuff Leak Test †

1. Assess the patient to ensure there is spontaneous efforts when disconnected from the ventilator
2. Suction the mouth / upper airway with Yankauer
3. Deflate ET Tube cuff
4. Briefly occlude the ET Tube
5. Positive Result: Patient can breathe around occluded ET tube
6. Negative Result: Pt cannot breathe around tube, suspect laryngeal edema

† From Sharar S: Weaning and extubation are not the same, ***Respiratory Care***, Vol. 40, pp.239-43, 1995.

There are several variations to the Cuff Leak test, including leaving the patient on the ventilator, placing it on a Volume mode of ventilation, performing steps 2-3 above, and then watching graphics and returned VT for a notable leak. In this way you can roughly measure the leak.

Extubation Procedure

Equipment Needed:

- Manual resuscitation bag with reservoir for 100% F_IO_2 with mask
- Oxygen source
- Oxygen mask or cannula (hooked up and running)
- High-volume suction source and equipment (appropriately sized catheter, large bore oral suction device)
- Oral and pharyngeal airways
- Reintubation equipment (if needed)
- A 10 cc syringe (for cuff deflation)
- Disposable "Chuck" / towel / pad

Procedure:

- Choose an appropriate time of the day (preferably AM) and not during shift change.
- Explain the procedure to the patient.
- Consider removal of NG/OG tube simultaneously with ET tube.
- Monitor patient throughout and after procedure (EKG, SpO_2).
- Sit patient in semi- or high Fowler's position.
- Pre-oxygenate patient with 100% F_IO_2.
- Suction the mouth and pharynx.
- Give large breath with hold as the cuff is being deflated to force secretions above the cuff (repeat until clear).
- Loosen the tape or ET Tube holder.
- Instruct patient to cough as ET tube is being removed (or hyperinflate patient).
- Remove tube (including OG/NG if appropriate) quickly and smoothly as pt. coughs.
- Instruct the patient to cough directly after the ET tube is removed.
- Have patient speak a word or two.
- Administer the same (or slightly higher) F_IO_2 as prior to extubation.
- Auscultate for BS, auscultate throat for stridor
- Encourage the patient to take deep breaths and cough.
- Monitor the patient closely.
- Obtain ABG after 1 hour (optional).

Discontinuation

Post-Extubation Care

Patients should be assessed immediately following extubation, both initially and then periodically (at least several times). Systematic assessment should minimally include:

- Ask patient to cough
- Ask patient to say a few words (mental status, vocal cord function)
- Auscultate (lung fields and throat)
- Check vitals (HR, RR, BP, SpO2)
- Check WOB (diaphoresis, paradoxical breathing)

If Stridor is present, consider:

- Cool aerosol by mask (supplemental O2 as needed)
- Nebulized racemic epinephrine (2-3 unit dosages may ne necessary)
- Heliox (80/20 or 70/30) delivered via NRB mask
- Concurrent steroid administration (IV)
- If Stridor is accompanied by diminished breath sounds and significant WOB, consider immediate reintubation

Reintubation Criteria

1. Consider brief trial of NPPV when clinically appropriate (see NPPV chapter). Extubation failure is considered if:

RR	> 35 breaths/min or < 6 breaths/min
$\dot{V}_E$	>10 L/min
HR	Tachycardia (>100beats/min) Bradycardia (< 60 beats/min)
BP	Hypotension (BPsys < 90 mmHg) Hypertension (BPsys >170 mmHg) or↑ > 20 mmHg ↑ baseline
ECG	New arrhythmias & ischemia

Common causes for extubation failure: Upper airway obstruction, inability to protect the airway, inability to remove secretions.

Note: Extubation failure can occur for reasons distinct from discontinuation failure.

Make It Your Own

Notes Page

Notes Page

A Appendix / Index

CONTENTS

Abbreviations/Terms A-2

AARC Clinical Practice Guideline Summaries

Capnography/Capnometry during Mechanical Ventilation A-4

Endotracheal Suctioning of Mechanically Ventilated Adults and Children with Artificial Airways A-5

Humidification during Invasive and Non-Invasive Mechanical Ventilation A-6

In-Hospital Transport of the Mechanically Ventilated Patient A-7

Removal of the Endotracheal Tube A-8

Index A-10

Abbreviations

AARC	American Association of Respiratory Care
A/C	Assist/control
ACCP	American College of Chest Physicians
ADH	Anti-diuretic hormone
ABG	Arterial blood gas
APRV	Airway pressure release ventilation
APV	Adaptive pressure ventilation
ARDS	Adult respiratory distress syndrome
ASV	Adaptive support ventilation
ATC	Automatic tube compensation
BiPAP	Bi-level positive airway pressure
BP	Blood pressure
BPD	Bronchopulmonary dysplasia
BPdia	Diastolic blood pressure
BPsys	Systolic blood pressure
B-P	Broncho-pleural
BSA	Body surface area
CABG	Coronary artery bypass graph
CaO_2	Arterial oxygen content
$Ca\text{-}\bar{v}O_2$	Arterial –mixed venous O_2 content difference
Ccw	Compliance of the chest wall
Cdyn	Dynamic compliance
CF	Conversion factor
CI	Cardiac index
CL	Compliance of the lung
CLT	Compliance of the lung and thorax
cm H_2O	Centimeters of water
CNS	Central nervous system
CO	Cardiac output
CO	Carbon monoxide
COPD	Chronic obstructive pulmonary disease
CPAP	Continuous positive airway pressure
CPG	Clinical Practice Guideline
CPP	Cerebral perfusion pressure
Cstat	Static compliance
Ctubing	Compliance of the tubing
CV	Cardiovascular
CVA	Cerebrovascular accident
CVP	Central venous pressure
CXR	Chest x-ray
E	Expiration
ECMO	Extracorporeal membrane oxygenation
EKG	Electrocardiogram
EPAP	Expiratory positive airway pressure
et	End-tidal
ET	Endotracheal
f	Frequency (ventilator rate)
FIO_2	Fraction of inspired oxygen
FRC	Functional residual capacity
F-T	Flow-time
GI	Gastrointestinal
Hgb	Hemoglobin
HME	Heat moisture exchanger
HR	Heart rate
I	Inspiration
ICP	Intracranial pressure
I:E	Inspiratory/expiratory ratio
IPAP	Inspiratory positive airway pressure
IRV	Inverse ratio ventilation
J	Joule
JVD	Jugular vein distention
kg	Kilogram
LBW	Low birth weight
LIP	Lower inflection point
LOC	Level of consciousness
LV	Left ventricle
MAP	Mean arterial pressure
MDI	Metered dose inhaler
MIF	See PImax
MIP	See PImax
mmHg	millimeters of mercury
MV	Mechanical ventilation
NIF	See PImax
NO	Nitric oxide
NPPV	Noninvasive positive pressure ventilation
O_2	Oxygen
O_2ER	Oxygen extraction ratio
P	Pressure
$PA\text{-}aO_2$	Alveolar-arterial oxygen partial pressure difference
$PaCO_2$	Partial pressure of arterial carbon dioxide
P-ACV	Pressure-assist/control ventilation
PAPD	Pulmonary artery diastolic pressure
Palv	Alveolar pressure
PAMP	Pulmonary artery mean pressure
PaO_2	Partial pressure of arterial oxygen

PAO_2	Partial pressure of alveolar oxygen
PAOP	Pulmonary artery occlusion pressure
PAP	Pulmonary artery pressure
Paug	Pressure augmentation
PAV	Proportional assist ventilation
Paw	Airway pressure
$\overline{P}aw$	Mean airway pressure
Pawo	Pressure at airway opening
PASP	Pulmonary artery systolic pressure
PAWD	Pulmonary artery wedge pressure
PCWP	Pulmonary capillary wedge pressure
PB	Barometric pressure
PBW	Predicted body weight
PEEP	Positive end-expiratory pressure
pH	Negative log of hydrogen ion concentration
PIE	Pulmonary interstitial emphysema
PImax	Maximal inspiratory pressure
PIP	Peak inspiratory pressure
P-IRV	Pressure-inverse ratio ventilation
PIT	Intrathoracic pressure
P-MMV	Pressure-mandatory minute ventilation
PMI	Point of maximal impulse
PP	Pulse pressure
Ppl	Intrapleural pressure
Ppeak	Peak inspiratory pressure
PPHN	Persistent pulmonary hypertension of the newborn
Pplat	Inspiratory plateau pressure
PPV	Positive pressure ventilation
PRVC	Pressure regulated volume control
P-SIMV	Pressure-synchronized intermittent mandatory ventilation
PSV	Pressure support ventilation
$PtcO_2$	Transcutaneous partial pressure of oxygen
PV	Pressure ventilation
$P\overline{v}O_2$	Partial pressure of oxygen in mixed venous blood
PVR	Pulmonary vascular resistance
Qs/Qt	Physiological shunt
Raw	Airway resistance
RHF	Right heart failure
ROP	Retinopathy of prematurity
RR	Spontaneous respiratory rate
SaO_2	Saturation of arterial oxygen
SCCM	Society of Critical Care Medicine
SpO_2	Saturation of arterial oxygen by pulse oximeter
$S\overline{v}O_2$	Saturation of oxygen in mixed venous blood
SVR	Systemic vascular resistance
TE	Expiratory time
T-E	Tracheo-esophageal
TGI	Tracheal gas insufflation
TI	Inspiratory time
Ttot	Total cycle time
UAC	Umbilical artery catheter
UIP	Upper inflection point
UO	Urinary output
V	Volume
$\dot{V}$	Flow
VA	Alveolar volume
$\dot{V}A$	Alveolar ventilation
V-ACV	Volume-assist/control ventilation
VAPS	Volume assured pressure support
VCO_2	Volume of carbon dioxide production
VD	Deadspace volume
ΞD	Deadspace ventilation
VD/VT	Deadspace/tidal volume ratio
$\dot{V}E$	Minute ventilation
$\dot{V}Emech$	Minute ventilation mechanical
$\dot{V}Espont$	Minute ventilation spontaneous
VILI	Ventilator-induced lung injury
V-IRV	Volume-inverse ratio ventilation
V-MMV	Volume-mandatory minute ventilation
$\dot{V}O_2$	Volume of oxygen consumption
VPC	Variable pressure support
V-P	Volume-pressure (curve)
VS	Volume support
V-SIMV	Volume-synchronized intermittent mandatory ventilation
VT	Tidal volume
Vtubing	Volume loss to tubing
V/Q	Ventilation/perfusion ratio
WOB	Work of breathing
VV	Volume ventilation

Capnography/Capnometry during Mechanical Ventilation[1,2] (AARC CPG)	
Indications • Verification of Artificial Airway Placement: All intubations MUST be confiromed by some form of $PETCO_2$ measurement • Assessment of Pulmonary Circulation and Respiratory Status: May be quicker than pulse oximetry in pts with lung disease, monitors adequacy of pulmonary, systemic, and coronary blood flow, and in screening for a pulmonary emboli • Optimization of Mechanical Ventilation: continuous monitoring of ventilator and circuit functional status, helps evaluate efficiency of ventilation, severity of disease, V/Q during ILV, and monitoring of inspired CO2 when therapeutically administered. • Evaluation of capnogram: May be useful in detecting rebreathing of CO2, obstructive disease, NMBA, and effectiveness of compressions during CPR. **Contraindications**: None	**Hazards / Complications** • ↑ V_D, • ↑ weight on artificial airway or line **Monitoring** • Ventilatory variables: V_T, f, PEEP, I/E, PIP, FIO_2 • Hemodynamic variables: BP (sys & pulm), CO, shunt, V/Q imbalances **Frequency:** PRN, during intubation **Limitations** • Is not a substitute for • assessing $PaCO_2$ • Reliability may be affected by: resp. gas mixture, RR, Freon, secretions/condensate, filters, leaks, low Cardiac Output or V_T.

1. Evaluation of CO_2 in respiratory gases on MV patients.
2. Adapted from AARC Clinical Practice Guideline: Capnography / Capnometry during Mechanical Ventilation: 2011, Respiratory Care, Vol. 56, #4, 2011
3. Low Cardiac Output may negate its use for this indication.

Endotracheal Suctioning of Mechanically Ventilated Adults and Children * † (AARC CPG)	

Indications
• Maintain airway patency
• Obtain sputum specimen
• Remove accumulated secretions as evidenced by:
  • Coarse crackles over trachea
  • Sawtooth pattern on Flow-Volume Loop
  • ABG deterioration
  • Acute respiratory distress
  • Suspected aspiration
  • Ineffective cough
  • Vent changes (↑ PIP in volume modes, ↓ V_T in pressure modes)
  • Visible secretions in airway
  • Suspected aspiration
 	
Contraindications
Relative: Adverse reaction or worsening clinical condition from the procedure.
 	
Frequency: Only when clinically indicated to maintain airway patency
	Hazards/Complications
	• Atelectasis
	• Bronchospasm/constriction
	• Cardiac arrhythmia/arrest
	• Hemorrhage/bleeding
	• Hypo/hypertension
	• Hypoxia/hypoxemia
	• ↑ ICP
	• Infection (patient or caregiver)
	• Interruption of MV
	• Mucosal trauma
	• Saline instillation may result in:
	• Excessive cough, ↓ SaO_2, Bronchospasm, Dislodgement of biofilm, pain, anxiety, dyspnea, tachycardia, ↑ ICP
	
	Monitoring
	ABGs/SaO_2, BS, cough effort, CV parameters (BP, HR, EKG), ICP, RR and pattern, skin color, sputum prod (color, volume, consistency, odor), ventilator parameters (PIP, Pplat, VT, graphics, FIO_2).

* A component of bronchial hygiene therapy involving the mechanical aspiration of pulmonary secretions from a patient with an artificial airway.

† Adapted from the AARC Clinical Practice Guideline: Endotracheal Suction of Mechanically Ventilated Adults and Children with Artificial Airways, ***Respiratory Care***, Vol. 55, #6, 2010.

Humidification during Invasive and Noninvasive Mechanical Ventilation (AARC CPG)

Indication

Mandatory when mechanically ventilated, with ET Tube or Tracheostomy, but optional with NPPV

Contraindication

None except HME when:

- Body temperature < 32°C, concurrent aerosol therapy, expired V_T < 70% of delivered V_T, spont $\dot{V}_E$ > 10 L/min, thick, copious, or bloody secretions, with low VT strategies (ARDS, etc.)
- Do not use HME with NPPV with large mask leaks

Monitoring

Check: alarm settings (41ºC at highest) (HR), humidifier temp setting (HR), inspired gas temp (37°C at the wye) (HR), water level and feed system (HR), sputum quantity and consistency

Remove condensate in circuit

Replace HMEs contaminated with secretions

Frequency:

Continuous during gas therapy

Hazards/Complications

- Burns (patient or caregiver) (HH)
- Electrical shock (HH)
- Hypo/hyperthermia
- Hypoventilation (HME → ↑VD)
- ↑ Resistive WOB through humidifier
- Infection (nosocomial)
- Tracheal lavage (pooled condensate or overfilling) (HH)
- Underhydration (mucous impaction or plugging of airways → air-trapping, hypoventilation, ↑ WOB
- Ventilator malperformance: pooled condensate → ↑ airway pressures or asynchrony with patient (HH)
- HME → ineffective low pressure alarm during disconnection
- Pt-Vent dyssynchrony due to pooled condensation (HH)

Clinical Goal

Humidified and warmed inspired gases without hazards or complications.

1) Adapted from AARC Clinical Practice Guideline: Humidification during Invasive and Noninvasive Mechanical Ventilation, ***Respiratory Care***, Vol. 57, #5, 2012.

HH = heated humidity, HME = heat moisture exchanger

In Hospital Transport of the Mechanically Ventilated Patient [1] (AARC CPG)	
Indications Following a careful evaluation of the risk-benefit ratio ***Contraindications*** • All members of transport team are not present.. • *Inability during transport to:* Adequately monitor CV status • Maintain acceptable hemodynamic performance • Maintain airway control • Provide adequate O_2 and ventilation ***Monitoring*** Same as during stationary care. *Continuous:* EKG, HR, BP (if invasive line), SpO_2 *Intermittent:* BS, RR, BP (no invasive line), PIP, VT	***Hazards/Complications*** • Accidental extubation or removal of IV access due to movement • CV instability • Equipment failure • Hyperventilation (manual ventilation) • Inadvertent disconnection of IVs or MV support • Loss of O_2 supply • Loss of PEEP/CPAP • Position changes causing ↓ BP, ↓ PaO_2, and/or ↑ $PaCO_2$ • VAP ***Assessment of Need:*** Risk vs. benefit ***Assessment of Outcome:*** Safe arrival ***Infection Control:*** Universal Precautions, disinfection of equip between patients, CDC recommendations for TB risk.

1) Adapted from AARC Clinical Practice Guideline: In-Hospital Transport of the Mechanically Ventilated Patient, ***Respiratory Care***, Vol. 47, #6, 2002.

Removal of the Endotracheal Tube - 2007* (AARC CPG)	
Indications • Airway control no longer necessary and patient is able to maintain patent airway & adequate spontaneous ventilation (i.e. adequate neuro drive, muscle strength, cough) • Artificial airway obstruction (not able to be cleared rapidly) • Discontinuance of further medical care **Contraindications**: No absolute **Hazards/Complications** • **Hypoxemia** (aspiration, atelectasis, bronchospasm, hypoventilation, laryngospasm, low O_2, pulmonary edema) • **Hypercapnia** (bronchospasm, excessive WOB, muscle weakness, upper airway edema) • **Death** (discontinuance of medical care)	**Assessment of Readiness** Artificial airway no longer needed as indicated by reversal of cause, adequate spontaneous ventilation and meet readiness criteria: • ***Maintain adequate PaO_2:*** $PaO_2/F_IO_2 > 150\text{-}200$, • PEEP ≤ 5-8 cm H_2O and • $FIO_2 \leq 0.4\text{-}0.5$ • Maintain appropriate pH > 7.25 and $PaCO_2$ • Cthorax > 25 mL/cmH_2O • f < 35/min (adult) • Modified CROP ≥ 0.1-0.15 mL.mmHg/breaths/min/mL/kg • MVV > 2x$\dot{V}E$ (resting) • NIP > - 20-30 cm H_2O • O_2 cost of breathing < 15% total • P0.1 < 6 cm H_2O • PEF ≥ 60 L/min • RSBI ≤ 105 (modified RSBI ≤ 8-11 breaths/min.mL.kg) • SMIP > 57.5 • Successful SBT (30-120 min) with low CPAP (5 cmH_2O) or low PS (5-7 cmH_2O) (i.e., adequate respiratory pattern, gas exchange, hemo stability and comfort) • VC > 10 mL/kg (ideal) • $V_D/V_T < 0.6$ • $\dot{V}_E$ (spont) < 10 L/min • WOB < 0.8 J/L.

(continued from previous page)	
Assessment of Outcome/ Monitoring Assess/monitor: ABGs, adequate spontaneous ventilation & oxygenation, airway patency, chest X-ray, complications, hemodynamics, neuro status, VS, WOB Note: Attentive monitoring, prompt ID of respiratory distress and maintaining patent airway is essential. **Infection Control** Follow CDC Standard Precautions	**Resolution of need for airway protection:** Adequate airway protective reflexes Easily managed secretions Normal consciousness **Other Considerations** Electrolytes Hemodynamics Nutrition Prophylactic meds (lidocaine, steroids) Reintubation need Risk factors Upper airway obstruction/ edema

* Adapted from AARC Clinical Practice Guideline: Removal of the Endotracheal Tube – 2007 Revision & Update, ***Respiratory Care***, Vol. 52, #1, 2007.

Index

A

A-a Gradient 7-4, 7-6
a/A Ratio 7-5, 7-6
AARC Clinical Practice Guidelines
  Capnography/Capnometry during Mechanical Ventilation A-4
  Endotracheal Suctioning of Mechanically Ventilated Adults and Children A-5
  Humidification during Mechanical Ventilation A-6
  In Hospital Transport of the Mechanically Ventilated Patient A-7
  Removal of the Endotracheal Tube A-8
Abbreviations A-2
ABG. See Arterial Blood Gases
ACCP Consensus Conference: Mechanical Ventilation 1-9
ACCP Discontinuation/Weaning Guidelines 12-15
Acid-base. See Arterial Blood Gases
  Equations 7-2
Acute Respiratory Distress Syndrome. See Mean Airway Pressure
Acute Respiratory Failure 1-3
  Differentials 1-5
  Invasive Ventilation Indications 1-4
Adaptive Pressure Ventilation 3-29. See also Pressure-Regulated Volume Control
Adaptive Support Ventilation 3-35
Adaptive Tidal Volume Support 3-35. See Adaptive Support Ventilation
Air Trapping. See Auto-PEEP
Air-Trapping 6-35
Airway Obstruction 5-11
  Causes, Signs & Symptoms 11-2
Airway Occlusion Pressure 7-14
Airway Pressure Release Ventilation 3-17
Airway Pressures. See Mean Airway Pressure
Airway Resistance
  Changes in 5-11, 6-38
  Equation 7-15
  Methods to Reduce 5-11
Alarms (initial, limits, problems) 4-16
Alveolar. See also Recruitment (Alveolar)
  Air Equation 7-5
  Oxygen Tension 7-5
  Pressure 2-7
  Ventilation 7-10
  Volume 7-10
American-European Consensus Conference
Anion gap 7-2
APRV 3-17
ARDS 10-2
  Alternative Techniques 10-7
  Berlin definition 10-2
  Diagnostic Criteria: 10-2
  Initial Settings 10-5
  Inspiratory Flow 4-13
  Management 10-6
  Phases 10-3
  Strategies 10-4–10-6
ARDSnet Protocol 10-8
Arterial/Alveolar O2 Tension 7-5
Arterial Blood Gases
  Mixed Venous 5-6
  Normal Values 5-6

Ventilator-Based Causes 11-12
Arterial Blood Pressure
Mean 7-23
Arterial CO2 Tension 7-6
Arterial- (mixed) Venous O2 Content Difference 7-6
Arterial- (mixed) Venous O2 Tension Difference 7-6
Arterial O2 Content 7-7
Artificial Airway
Dyssynchrony 8-23
Assist/Control
Pressure 3-13
Volume 3-7
Asthma 10-13
National Asthma Education Guideline 10-16
Near-Fatal 10-17
ASV 3-35
Asynchrony. See Dyssynchrony
Atelectasis
Causes, Signs & Symptoms 11-2
ATPS to BTPS 7-27
Autoflow
Automatic Tube Compensation 3-39
Automode 3-41
Auto-PEEP 2-11, 4-14, 6-51, 11-3
Causees, Signs & Symptoms 11-3
Dyssynchrony 8-23
Measuring 2-11, 11-5
Methods to Reduce 11-6
Treating 8-17
a-vDO2 7-6

B

Bag & Valve Mask Ventilation 8-4
Base
Deficit 7-2
Excess 7-2
Bicarbonate Correction of pH 7-3
Bilevel 3-20. See also Airway Pressure Release Ventilation
Bivent 3-19
Bi-Vent. See also Airway Pressure Release Ventilation
Body Surface Area Equations 7-26
Bohr Equation 7-12
Boyle's Law 7-27
BP Fistula
Management of 10-19
Bronchopleural Fistula
Management of 10-19
BSA 7-26
Burns and Smoke Inhalation
Management of 10-21

C

CaO2 5-6, 5-7, 7-7
Capnography
Capography/Capnometry During Mechanical Ventilation A-4
Cardiac
Index 7-22
Management of (Disorders) 10-26
Output 7-22
Cardiovascular Effects of PPV 11-14
Ca-vO2 7-6
CcO2 7-7
Charles' Law 7-27
Chest Trauma 10-35
CHF

Management of 10-26
Chronic Obstructive Pulmonary Disease. See COPD
Circuit Compressible Volume 4-5
Compliance
Changes in 6-41
Dynamic 5-10, 7-18
Equations 7-16
Tubing 4-5
Congestive Heart Failure
Management of 10-26
Continuous Distending Pressure. See CPAP
Continuous Mechanical Ventilation. See V-ACV
Continuous Positive Airway Pressure. See CPAP
Continuous Positive Pressure Breathing. See CPAP
COPD
Inspiratory Flow 4-13
Management of 10-23
NPPV Management 9-9
Tube Compensation 3-39
Coronary Artery Perfusion Pressure 7-22
CPAP 3-43
Weaning (Abrupt) 12-12
Weaning (Gradual) 12-14
CPP 7-22
CROP 7-21
Cstat 7-17
Cuff Leak Test 12-24
Cycle Dysynchrony 8-27

D

Dalton's Law 7-27
Deadspace
Mechanical 2-16, 4-5
Dead Space
Ventilation 7-11
Volume 7-11
Deadspace/Tidal Volume Ratio 7-12
Discontinuation. See Weaning
Assessment 12-3
Cardiovascular Assessment 12-8
Definitions 12-2
Electrolyte Assessment 12-8
Metabolic Assessment 12-8
Miscellaneous Factors 12-11
Monitoring of Success/Failure 12-21
Neurologic Assessment 12-9
Nutritional Assessment 12-9
Pharmacological Assessment 12-9
Predictive Indices 12-3
Renal Assessment 12-11
Discontinuation Failure
Common Causes for 12-22
Discontinuation Methods 12-12
Distress
Patient Problems 5-4
Ventilator Problems 5-5
DO2 7-8
DO2I 7-8
DO2 - VO2 7-8
Drug Overdose
Management of 10-29
Duration of a Cylinder 7-29
Duration of a Liquid System 7-29
Dynamic Compliance 7-18
Dyssynchrony 5-17, 8-22
Cycle 8-27
Expiratory (Demand) Valves 8-24
Flow 8-27
Humidifiers 8-24

Mode 8-26
Trigger 8-25

E

Edi (NAVA) 3-37
Emergent Airway Management
Intubation Procedure 8-2
End Expiratory Pause 2-11
End-tidal CO2 Detector 8-3
Equation of Motion 7-19
Esophageal Detector Device 8-3
ET Tube. See also Intubation/Extubation
Removal of (AARC CPG) A-8
Suctioning (AARC CPG) A-5
Excessive (Active) Exhalation 6-43
Expiratory (Demand) Valves
Dyssynchrony 8-24
Expiratory Hold 2-11
Expiratory Sensitivity 4-14
Expiratory Time 2-9
Extubation 12-24
Assessment for Removal 12-24
Failure 12-26
Post-Extubation Care 12-26
Procedure 12-25
Removal of the Endotracheal Tube A-8, A-9

F

Fick Equation 7-22
Fick's Law of Diffusion 7-27
Fighting the Ventilator. See also Dyssynchrony
Potential Causes 5-17
FIO2 2-13
Estimation 7-6
Initial Setting 4-10
Flow Dysynchrony 8-27
Flow Rate 4-13
Flow Starvation 6-49
Flow-Time Waveform 6-9
Flow-Volume Loop 6-14
Flow Waveforms 4-13
Frequency 4-7
Calculating New Rate 4-7
f / VT 7-20

G

Gas laws 7-27
Gay-Lussac's Law 7-27
Graham's Law of Diffusion Coefficient 7-27
Graphic Waveforms
Abnormals by Problem 6-35
Abnormals by Waveform Type 6-26
by Waveform Type 6-16
Types Of 6-4

H

Head Trauma 10-37
Helium/Oxygen (He/O2) Flow Conversion 7-28
Henderson-Hasselbach Equation 7-3
Hepatic Effects of PPV 11-14
Humidification 2-16
during Ventilation (AARC CPG) A-6
Initial Setting 4-15
Switching to heated humidity 4-15
Humidifiers
Dyssynchrony 8-24

Hypercapnia
  permissive 8-10
Hypercapnic Respiratory Failure 1-3
Hyperventilation
  Causes of 5-8
Hyperventilation therapy 1-2
Hypoventilation
  Causes of 5-8
Hypoxemic respiratory failure 1-3

I

Ideal Body Weight (IBW) 7-27
I:E Ratio 2-10, 2-17–2-20
  Initial Settings 4-12
  Inspiratory Time Chart 4-12
Impending Respiratory Failure 1-2
Indications for Ventilatory Support
  Parameters Used to Determine Ventilatory Need 1-8
Infection 11-15
Inspiratory Assist. See Airway Pressure Release Ventilation
Inspiratory Cycle Off 4-14
Inspiratory:Expiratory Ratio. See I: E Ratio
Inspiratory Flow 2-12
Inspiratory Flow Rate 4-13
Inspiratory Flow Waveform 2-12, 4-13
Inspiratory Hold (Pause) 2-7, 2-11
Inspiratory Pressure 4-8
  Peak 2-6
  Plateau Pressure 2-7
Inspiratory Time 2-9
  Initial Setting 4-11
Intubation
  Checklist 8-2
  Procedure 8-2
Inverse Ratio Ventilation 8-21

L

Law of LaPlace 7-28
Leaks (checking for) 5-15
Left Ventricular Stroke Work 7-23
Left Ventricular Stroke Work Index 7-23
Liberation 12-2
Loops 6-4, 6-11
  Abnormal Flow-Volume 6-33
  Abnormal Volume-Pressure 6-30
  Flow-Volume 6-24
  Volume-Pressure 6-22
Lung Compliance Equations 7-16
Lung Failure 1-3
Lung Protective Strategies 11-11

M

Mandatory Minute Ventilation
  Pressure 3-23
  Volume 3-11
MAP. See Mean Airway Pressure; See Mean Arterial Blood Pressure
  Confusion in terms 2-7
Maximal Inspiratory Pressure 7-19
Mean Airway Pressure 2-7, 7-20, 8-19
Mean Arterial Blood Pressure 7-23
Mean Pulmonary Artery Pressure 7-23
Mechanical Deadspace 2-16, 4-5
Mechanical Ventilation
  Contraindications 1-3
  Indications 1-2, 1-4–1-5
  Objectives 1-9

Parameters to determine need 1-8
Types 2-2
Mechanics Equations 7-14
Minute Ventilation (or Volume) 2-4, 4-3, 4-4, 7-12
MIP 7-19
Mixed Venous O2 Saturation 7-9
Mode Dysynchrony 8-26
Modes of Ventilation 3-2
Breath Types 3-1
Classification 3-1
Definition 3-1
Mode Key 3-5
Summary Use Chart 3-45
MVV 1-8
Myocardial Infarction
Management of 10-26

N

National Asthma Education Guidelines 10-16
NAVA. See Neurally Adjusted Ventilatory Assist
Near-Fatal Asthma 10-17
Neurally Adjusted Ventilatory Assist 3-37
Neurological Effects of PPV 11-14
Neuromuscular Disorders
Management of 10-30
NIP 7-19
Non-Invasive. See NPPV
Non-Invasive Positive Pressure Ventilation. See NPPV
NPPV 9-1, 12-14
Acute Care 9-2, 9-7
Choosing an Interface 9-13
Choosing a Ventilator 9-12
Chronic Care 9-9
Clinical benefits of 9-7
Complications of 9-8
Contraindications to Chronic Use 9-9
Criteria for stopping 9-11
Discontinuation 12-14
Dysynchrony 9-10
Goals of 9-7
Humidity 9-10
Indications by Disease 9-4, 9-9
Management 9-10
Predicting Success 9-7
Selection and Exclusion Criteria for 10-23
Treatment Failure 9-7
Weaning 9-10
Nutritional Effects of PPV 11-14

O

O2. See Oxygen
Obstructive Sleep Apnea
NPPV Management 9-9
OI 7-8
Open Lung Approach 11-11
Over-Distension 6-45, 11-10
Minimizing 11-12
Oxygen
Blending ratios 7-28
Consumption 7-7
Consumption Index 7-7
Content 7-7
Delivery 7-8
Delivery Index 7-8
Demand 7-7
Entrainment Ratios 7-30

Extraction Ratio (ER) 7-8
Initial Setting 4-10
Reserve 7-8
Saturation (mixed venous) 7-9
Supply 7-8
Tank Duration 7-29
Toxicity 11-7
Transport 7-8
Oxygenation
at the Lungs 5-7
at the Tissues 5-7
Determinants of 2-20
Failure 1-3
Methods for Improving 8-12–8-21
Quick Estimates 8-11
Ratio 7-9
Oxygenation, Optimizing
APRV 3-17
Bilevel 3-20
Bi-Vent 3-19
Oxygen Index 7-8

P

P0.1 7-14
PA-aO2 1-8, 5-7
PA-aO2 / PaO2 5-7, 7-9
Palv 2-7
PaO2 1-8, 5-7
PAO2 7-5
PaO2 (based on age) 7-9
PaO2 / FIO2 1-8, 5-7, 7-9
PaO2 / PAO2 7-5
PaO2/PAO2 5-7
PAO2 Targets 4-10
Parameters
Expiratory hold 2-11
Expiratory time 2-9
Frequency 2-5
I:E Ratio 2-10
Inspiratory Flow 2-12
Inspiratory Flow Waveform 2-12
Inspiratory pause 2-11
Inspiratory Time 2-9
Mean Airway Pressure 2-7
Minute Ventilaton 2-4
Peak Inspiratory Pressure 2-6
PEEP 2-8
Plateau Pressure 2-7
Rate 2-5
Tidal Volume 2-4
Partial Obstruction 6-44
Patient Calculations 7-26
Patient Distress (Sudden) 5-3
Patient Positioning 8-20.
Patient-Ventilator Asynchrony
Common Signs 8-22
Potential Causes 5-17
PAV 3-30
Pa-vO2 7-6
Paw 2-7, 7-20
Peak Inspiratory Pressure 2-6, 4-8
PEEP 2-8, 4-9, 7-17, 8-13. See also Auto-PEEP
Applied 8-17
Beneficial Effects of Appropriate PEEP 8-13
Hemodynamics of 8-18
Initial Setting 4-9, 8-14
Measuring and Monitoring 8-18
Optimal 2-8, 8-15

Potential Adverse Effects of 8-13
Ranges 8-14
treating auto-PEEP 8-17, 11-6
Types 2-8
Perfusion/Hemodynamic Monitoring Equations 7-22
Periodic Hyperinflation 2-15
Permissive Hypercapnia 8-10, 8-11
P/F ratio 7-6, 7-9
PI Max 1-8, 7-19
PIP 2-6
Plateau Pressure 2-7
Poiseuille"s law 7-30
Positioning (patient) 8-20
Positive End-Expiratory Pressure. See PEEP
Positive Pressure Ventilation
Selected Effects 11-14
Types 2-3
Post-Extubation Care 12-26
Post-Operative Patients
Management of 10-32
Ppeak 2-6
Pplat 2-7, 7-17
Predicted PaO2 (based on age) 7-9
Pressure-Regulated Volume Control 3-27
Pressure Support Ventilation 3-21
Pressure -Time Waveform 6-4
Pressure Ventilation 2-3
Determining VT Delivery 4-5
Factors Affecting Delivered VT 4-6
How To Set Pressure 4-5
Operating Principles 2-19
Vs. Volume Ventilation 2-3
Pressure Ventilation (Modes)
APRV 3-17
Assist/Control 3-13
Bi-Vent 3-19
MMV 3-23
PRVC 3-27
PSV 3-21
SIMV 3-15
Prophylactic Ventilatory Support 1-2
Proportional Assist Ventilation 3-30
Proportional Pressure Support 3-30
Proximal Airway Pressure. See Peak Inspiratory Pressure
PRVC 3-27
PTA 7-15
Pulmonary Artery Pressure
Mean 7-23
Pulmonary Capillary O2 Content 7-7
Pulmonary Vascular Resistance 7-23, 11-7
Pulmonary Vascular Resistance Index 7-24
Pulse Pressure 7-24
Pump Failure 1-3
PVR 7-23
PVRI 7-24

Q

QS/QT 1-8, 5-7

R

Rapid Shallow Breathing Index. See RSBI
Rate 4-7
Rate (Cycle) Asynchrony 6-48
Rate Pressure Product 7-24
Ratio Flow Factor 7-14
Raw 7-15
RE 7-9
Readiness Testing 12-2
Recruitment. See also PEEP (Optimal)
Recruitment (alveolar)

Sigh 2-15
Reintubation Criteria 12-26
Removal of the Endotracheal Tube A-8
Renal Effects of PPV 11-14
Respiration
External 5-7
Internal 5-7
Respiratory
Drive 11-7
Exchange Ratio 7-9
Failure 1-3
Index 7-9
Insufficiency 1-3
Quotient 7-9
Restrictive Disorders
NPPV Management 9-9
Restrictive Pulmonary Lung Disorders
Management of 10-34
Reynold's Number 7-30
RFF 7-14
RI 7-9
Right Ventricular Stroke Work 7-24
Right Ventricular Stroke Work Index 7-24
Rise Time 2-13
RPP 7-24
RQ 7-9
RR 7-9
RSBI 1-8, 7-20
RSBI Procedure 12-22
Rule of 8's 7-3

S

SaO2 1-8, 5-7
SBT 12-2, 12-12
Scalars 6-4
Abnormal Flow-Time 6-29
Abnormal Pressure-Time 6-26
Abnormal Volume-Time 6-28
Flow-Time 6-20
Pressure-Time 6-16
Volume-Time 6-18
Sensitivity 2-14, 4-14, 8-25
Inappropriate 6-50
Shunt Equation 7-25
Sigh 2-15
Simplified Weaning Index 7-21
SIMV. See Synchronized Intermittent Mandatory Ventilation
Smart Care Pressure Support 3-32
Smoke Inhalation (management) 10-21
SpO2 5-7
Spontaneous Breathing Trial 12-2, 12-12
Static Compliance 7-17. See also Compliance (5-10, 7-17)
5-10, 7-17
Stroke Volume 7-26
Stroke Volume Index 7-26
SvO2 7-9
SVR 7-26
SWI 7-21
Synchronized Intermittent Mandatory Ventilation
Pressure 3-15
Volume 3-9
Synchrony 8-22–8-27
NAVA (mode) 3-38
Synchrony Techniques
Neurally Adjusted Ventilatory Assist 3-37
Systemic Vascular Resistance 7-26
Systemic Vascular Resistance Index 7-26

T

T40 bicarbonate 7-4
TC 7-20
TE 2-9
Temperature Conversion 7-30
Terminal Discontinuation
TI 2-9
Tidal Volume 2-4, 2-17–2-20
  Calculating 4-4
  Factors Affecting 4-5–4-6
  Improperly Set (Concerns) 4-6
  Initial Setting 4-4
Time Constant 7-20
Tracheostomy (considerations for) 12-19
Transairway Pressure 7-15
Transport (intra-hospital) (AARC CPG) A-7
Trauma (Chest)
  Management of 10-35
Trauma (Head)
  Management of 10-37
Trigger Asynchrony 6-50
Trigger (Inspiratory) 4-14
Trigger Sensitivity 2-14
  Dyssynchrony 8-25
Troubleshooting
  Changes in Ventilator Parameters 5-13
Tube Compensation. See Automatic Tube Compensation
Tubing Compliance 4-5

V

VA 7-10
V-ACV 3-7–3-8, 3-9, 3-11
VAE. See Ventilatory Associated Events
VALI 11-10
VAP. See Ventilator Associated Events
VAPS 3-24
Variable Pressure Control. See Pressure-Regulated Volume Control
Variable Pressure Support
VC 7-21
VD 7-11
VDmech 2-16, 4-5
VD/VT 1-8
VD /VT ratio 7-12
VE 7-12
Venous O2 Content 7-7
Ventilation. See also Mechanival Ventilation
  Assessment of 5-8
  Changes in 5-8
Ventilation/Perfusion
  Imbalances 11-8
  Index 7-10
  Nomogram 7-13
  Ratio 7-13
Ventilator Assessment 5-12
Ventilator Associated Events 11-15
  Prevention 11-15
  VAP Bundle 11-15
Ventilator Associated Lung Injury 11-10
Ventilator Bundle 11-15
Ventilator Calculations 7-14
Ventilator Flow 7-14
Ventilator Induced Lung Injury
  Causes 11-10
  Ways to Minimize
Ventilator Leaks
  Checking for 5-15
Ventilator Management
  Improving Oxygenation 8-11
Ventilator Rate 2-5. See also Frequency

Needed for desired PaCO2 7-14
Ventilator Troubleshooting 5-3, 5-13
Ventilatory Capacity 12-2
Assessment of 5-9
Ventilatory Demand 12-2
Ventilatory Drive
Factors increasing or decreasing 12-7
Ventilatory Failure 1-3
Ventilatory Load
Assessment of 5-9
Ventilatory Mechanics
Assessment of 5-9
Changes in 5-10
Ventilatory Support
Clinical Parameters to determine ventilatory need 1-8
Contraindications 1-3
Full 2-2
Indications 1-2
Partial 2-2
Volume VS Pressure 2-3
VILI
See Ventilator Induced Lung Injury
Vital Capacity 7-21
VO2 7-7
VO2I 7-7
Volume-Assist/Control Ventilation 3-7
Volume-Assured Pressure Support 3-24
Volume Control Plus. See Pressure-Regulated Volume Control
Volume-Pressure Loop 6-11
Volume Support 3-33
Volume-Time Waveform 6-7
Volume Ventilation
Basic Operating Principles 2-17
Factors Affecting Delivered VT 4-5
Vs. Pressure Ventilation 2-3
Volume Ventilation (Modes)
Assist/Control 3-7
MMV 3-11
SIMV 3-9
VAPS 3-24
V/Q. See Ventilation/Perfusion
VQI 7-10
VS (Volume Support) 3-33

W

Waveforms. See Graphic Waveforms
Weaning 12-12, 12-23. See also Discontinuation
ACCP Guidelines 12-15
Assessment 12-3
Definitions 12-2
Equations 7-21
Failure 12-21
Inability to 12-2, 12-19
Methods 12-12
Predictive Indices 12-4
Weaning index 7-21
Winters Formula 7-4
Work of Breathing (WOB) 7-21, 11-8
Causes 11-8
Signs & Symptoms 11-8
Strategies to Reduce 11-9